HANDBOOK
FOR HOMOEOPATHY
DIGESTIVE TRACT REMEDIES

I0480115

J.V. MALLAPA RAJU

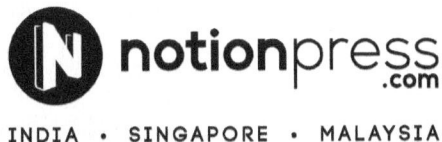

INDIA • SINGAPORE • MALAYSIA

Notion Press

No.8, 3rd Cross Street
CIT Colony, Mylapore
Chennai, Tamil Nadu – 600004

First Published by Notion Press 2020
Copyright © J.V. Mallapa Raju 2020
All Rights Reserved.

ISBN 978-1-64899-603-0

Dedicate to
Lord Sita Rama

CONTENTS

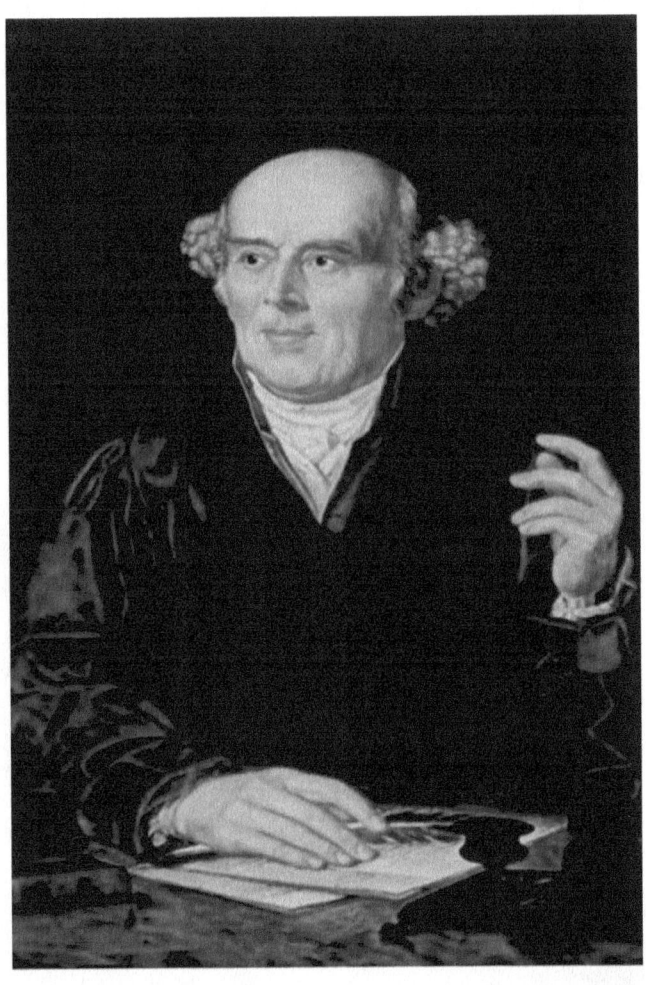

Samuel Christian Friedrich Hahnemann (1755 – 1843)

How an APPLE helped Newton to perceive the gravitational force of the earth "CINCHONA BARK" helped SAMUEL HAHNEMANN to establish the theory of HOMOEOPATHY "Similia Similibus Curantor"

AUTHOR'S NOTE

This is my second book after "Handbook for Homeopathy". While I was ending my earlier book I was thinking about, my next book's topic. And, started to revisit all the cases which I have attended.

In my last 35 years of practising homeopathy, I had a chance to address vivid types of cases. Some were chronic, and some of them were simple complaints. But all these had a common element, their digestive system. All patients who visited me had issues either due to poor functioning of their digestive system or by the mis-interpretation of one's body anatomy.

The one other cause which got highlighted in my research that due to the changes in our lifestyle, schedules and eating habits, has tampered our body clock so badly which lead people to develop issues like kidney stones, gall bladder stones, lesions in the stomach at an extreme level. The common symptoms like constipation, bloating, belching, heartburn etc., are observed even at a very young age.

Hence I started this book on unearthing the facts about 30+ foot long digestive tract, as a collation of my findings with bright patients that I came across and how I was able to help them in getting issues resolved.

While I was penning down the details, my main intent was to make one aware with the secrets of digestive system and to recommend, best and simple practices which can be followed by anyone even in their busiest of their times, so that they can retune their body clock and lead a healthy life.

(1ˢᵗEdition–2020)   J.V. MALLAPA RAJU

May Lord Sita Rama give you good health.
Oṃ sarvebhavantu sukhinaḥ sarvesantuni rāmayāḥ
sarvebhadrāṇi paśyantumāka ścidduḥkha bhāgbhaveta |
Oṃ śāntiḥ śāntiḥ śāntiḥ ||

APPEAL TO READERS

CHAPTER - 1

BASIC CONCEPT OF HOMOEOPATHY

Basic concept of treating **likes with likes** which are capable of producing symptoms in a healthy person also cure the likes those experienced in the patient remained undeveloped. The founder of modern system of Homoeopathic Treatment was a brilliant German physician **Dr. SAMUEL HAHNEMANN,** originally an allopath. During treatment with Allopathic medicines, he made the following observations:

Though the present symptoms were relieved, some new symptoms have come out in patients and were travelling below upwards and from surface to centre.

Further deep in the matter found that reasons are as under:

Medicines used being crude in nature they are palliating the present symptoms but bringing new symptoms.

Since medicines are having contrary symptoms, disease is travelling from below upwards and from surface to centre.

Using compound of medicines is also the reason for the manifestation of above order of symptoms.

To avoid bad prognosis of case, he thought that medicines are to be diluted thoroughly, single remedy to be given at a time and that relief of symptoms should be from top to bottom.

On further study Dr. Hahneman observed, as the medicines used in crude form, disease travelling from below upwards and from "surface to the centre".

As such he concluded that cure should be from above downwards and from centre to the surface and not vice versa, and wanted to seek ways and means to achieve this.

CONCEPTS OF HOMOEOPATHY AND ON THEIR DETAILS

- Similia Similibus Curantor – i.e. Likes cures the likes
- Cure should be from above downwards and from centre to surface
- Administration of Single remedy

Similia Similibus Curantor – i.e. Likes cures the likes

Cure of diseases quickly, safely, and effectively can be achieved, only with remedies which are capable of producing symptoms **Similar** to those existing in the patient. As per the therapeutic law of similarity, medicines should cure affections similar, or like unto those they produce.

Example:

While cutting an Onion (botanical name Allium Cepa), tears from eyes, burning and running of the nose is experienced which are similar to the symptoms that of compared with first day of common cold.

Hence medicine prepared from Onion (Allium Cepa) should give relief to the symptoms of first day common cold based on above concept. When the Homeo remedy prepared from Onion i.e. "Allium Cepa' in 30 potency administered is giving relief from symptoms of common cold.

In the above example, Onion (Allium cepa) is 'Similia' – symptoms of common cold i.e. running of nose and tears from the eyes, is 'Similibus' – 'Curantor' means cures those symptoms. Thus the theory "Similia Similibus Curantor" is proved.

Cure should be from above downwards and from centre to surface

When a remedy is administered, it should first give relief in the 'Mind' and later on to the body or give relief to the internal parts of the body i.e. Heart, Respiratory Tract, Stomach, Endocrinal glands etc. In addition, it should bring out toxins of the body from **Centre to the surface i.e. skin.** This remembers sweeping the house from within outwards and not vice versa. Body has tendency to sweep the toxins from within outwards, through urine, sweat etc. Hence medicine selected should assist the body to do this function effectively. **The basic system of treatment in Homoeopathy, is throwing out the disease from centre to surface.**

Example: In case of 'ASTHMA', keeping the etiological (route cause) factors being suppression of earlier skin symptoms for the manifestation of present disease i.e. ASTHMA, when Homoeopathic treatment is given the earlier suppressed skin symptoms in that case reappeared.

Administration of Single remedy

Dr. Hahnemann found

- Prescribing *different or combination of medicines,* against each part of the body or external applications for skin manifestations, are contrary to the principles of cure.
- Only a single remedy prepared with single material is to be administered and that medicine should cover all the symptoms of the patients. This can be achieved by 'PROVING' different materials thoroughly diluted on healthy human beings and not on animals as is done in Allopathy.

PROCESS OF PROVING

Proving is a system of eliciting symptoms after administration of a *diluted or potentized material* – prepared from vegetables/metals or salts etc. – on a **healthy man.** It is done on 8 to 10 healthy people who jot down the symptoms that have been experienced by each of them, in their own language. Now when the remedy prepared from such proved material administered to a patient, it is confirmed relief from the symptoms of the patient.

Recollect the example of 'ALLIUM CEPA' – (Onion) quoted earlier, i.e. justified the concept of 'SIMILIA SIMILIBUS CURANTOR'.

In the same process, materials in very a minute size, from Metals i.e – Gold, Silver, Iron, Zinc; Acids – Nitric Acid, Sulphuric Acid. Phosphoric Acid: Poisons – Snake poison, Bee poisons, etc. *proving is* done, and labelled with names accordingly. When the remedies so prepared are administered to patients depending upon the symptoms observed in each case of suffering by the patients, relief observed.

ASSUMPTIONS

Miasms and their influence on chronic diseases

Miasm is an agent that was passed down from generation to generation and a hereditary mechanism acting within the body. He postulated that miasms were mutations of partially cured diseases passed down from the earlier generations and that suppression of skin eruptions by allopathic treatment helped to fuel the Psoric miasm by *driving it underground* only to reappear in a chronic form in *later generations*.

As per Psora theory chronc diseases are caused or abetted by some constitutional dyscrasia, inherited or acquired, that lies dormant in the system. If a disease has been suppressed instead of cure, *especially if such suppression due to external applications*, it will rise not only to *constitutional symptoms*, but taint the entire organism, predisposing the system to many other diseases by lowering its power of resistance, as well as modifying from any other disease, the patient may afterwards suffer. First efforts, therefore, in treating any chronic disease, *must be directed to find out removing any original taint*, that may exist *so as to assess the clear picture or cure of the disease, that the patient comes to us for treatment*. (Aetiology i.e. background of the present complaint).

According to Hahnemann's Miasmic theory, the origin of all chronic diseases may be:

- **PSORIC** ... (Developed due to Suppression of skin eruptions)
- **SYCOTIC** ... (Developed due to Suppression of Gonorrhea)
- **SYPHILITIC**... (Diseases Developed due to Suppression of Syphilis)

As per modern times, the Miasmic Theory is in terms of our knowledge of the genetic code and the existence **"Deoxyribo Nucleic Acid (DNA)"** and **"Ribo Nucleic Acid (RNA),** which now known as they play a major part in hereditary characteristics.

Hahnemann's theory is rejected by many physicians claiming that his ideas were purely empirical and bore no relation to homoeopathy. *Whereas, the concept of miasms has been a revival in recent years* and has been broadened to include any illness although apparently cleared by treatment, leaves a residual effect, which may manifest itself in a chronic condition.

Hahnemann, in his notes of – THE CHRONIC DISEASES – stated:

Only three chronic miasms are (i) diseases caused, by themselves through **local symptoms,** and (ii) from which most, if not all, the chronic diseases originated, namely:

- **PSORA:**
- **SYPHILLIS:** (which he calls venereal chancre disease)
- **SYCOSIS:** (Figwart disease)
- **PSORA.** The chronic disease, which is at the foundation of the eruption of itch scabies, which he calls the latter, is the most important. **Psora is the oldest** miasmatic chronic disease known to us'. "Hahnemann stated that it was continual repeated fact that the non-venereal chronic diseases, after being time and again removed homoeopathically, always returned again in a more or less varied form with new symptoms, or reappeared annually.

- **PSORA** can also be taken as meaning 'evil thinking', **Sycosis** "evil operation **and**" Evil result" being **Syphillis.** Considered as '**Itch**' – Itch of the mind prominently – A clean mind do not **attract Psora** and, all its operations are clean, hence does not possess Sycosis so the result is bright finally does not possess the Syphillis constitution.

- The **PSORA** is the only fundamental route cause of all (chronic) diseases of a non-venereal nature. It is the mother of all diseases. Psora provided the fertile soil on which other miasms grow.

PSORA MAY BE RECOGNISED BY

- Mental and Physical irritability
- Fear, anxiety and restlessness
- Tendency to rashes, eruptions and catarrhal conditions
- Periodicity of complaint
- Susceptibility to parasitic infestation and fungal infection
- Delayed recovery from disease
- Failure to respond to selected remedies

A remedy which gives relief or antidotes the Psoric symptoms is an Anti-Psoric remedy. Similar is the case of an anti-Sycotic or anti-Syphilitic remedies.

The symptoms of anti-psoric miasm is well defined in the medicine "SULPHUR". In other words, by study of the remedy **"Sulphur"** one can get the idea of the miasm **PSORA**, completely, as all its mental and body symptoms are that of with Psoric background.

One or two doses of **Sulphur** are given, it anti-dotes most of the symptoms of Psora found. This is the reason to call it as **King of anti-Psoric miasm.**

However, it should not be construed that "Sulphur" remedy suit to all who are having Psoric symptoms.

SYCOSIS – OR THE FIG WART DISEASE

- It is a chronic venereal miasm due to suppression of gonorrheal discharge.
- Represented by warts, moles, and tumours, i.e. there is a general tendency towards overgrowths. Mentally Sycosis patient is a born criminal, revengeful and angry. He will never think twice before killing the person to whom he does not like. Unpredictable nature and will always do the most unpredictable things.

SYCOSIS IS RECOGNISED BY

- Anger
- Criminal bent up of mind
- Unpredictable and suspicious nature – keep agent on agent
- Self-condemnations
- Tendency for warts, tumors or overgrowths
- Humid and Progressive Asthma or respiratory ailments General relief from discharges

King of anti-scycotic remedy is 'Thuja as study of the remedy **Thuja** gives an idea of Sycotic miasm. As in the case of Sulphur if one or two **doses of Thuja** are given, it anti-dote most of the symptoms of Sycosis found in a patient and hence it is called **King of Sycotic miasm**. As in the case of **Sulphur**, it should not be construed that remedy "Thuja" suit to all who are having Sycotic symptoms, but should not depend only on Thuja when there are variations in the symptoms and should go to another remedy.

SYPHILLIS OR THE DESTRUCTIVE MIASM

The ultimate destructive venereal miasm due to suppression of syphilitic ulcer or bubo. Represented by punched out ulcers, with sloughing i.e. rotting of the tissues.

Mentally the patient is in rage. Syphilitic patient looses the most important things in life, and that is 'love for life' i.e. loose interest to live, depressive or may develop suicidal tendency.

SYPHILLIS IS RECOGNISED BY

- Rage
- Hate of life
- Slow, sullen stupid individuals
- Indurations (thickening of tissues) and ulcerations
- The periosteum and long bones especially involved
- Aggravation of all complaints during night time

King of anti-syphilitic remedy is 'Mercurius'. Study of Mercurius, projects Syphilitic miasm. One or two doses of Mercurius anti-dotes most of the symptoms of Syphilitic miasm found in a patient and this is why it is called king of Anti-syphilitic miasm.

PRECISELY THE SYMPTOMS OF MIASMS ARE AS UNDER

PSORA	SYCOSIS	SYPHILIS
Evil thinking	Evil application	Evil result
Mind very sharp & Intelligent	Mind – Suspicious– Wavering or Indecisive	Mind – Dull
Body: All functional disorders & skin mani-festations. Diseases pertai-ning to Digestive Tract	Body: Affects circulatory system, endocrinal glands muscular system, respiratory system and creates over growths, tumors, warts, rheumatism, Genito – Urinary tract diseases	Body Creates malignant ulcers, abscesses, malignant tumors, TuberculosisDiseases – of bones and TB or caries of bones

Physique: Tall and lean	Physique: Medium height and stout	Physique Dwarf and stout
Symptoms – Aggravation of During Day time – i.e sunrise to sunset	Aggravation of symptoms – During Day time – i.e. sunrise to sunset	< Of symptoms During Night time

Is it possible that **every Humanbeing** is restricted only to single Miasmatic Influence?

(A) No man on earth is **purely** – Psoric, Sycotic or Syphilitic i.e. may not possess only the symptoms of a particular miasm.

- In **Psoric** miasm stress on the mind is a must, thereby it becomes route cause for many a complaints. Hence Psora is a must, active, may be in a different degree, causing functional disorders. Without functional disorders, there is no possibility for disease, or other miasms. In other words, functional disorders may first paralyze endocrinal secretions (Glandular functions) which may in turn collapse of entire human body. Hence with Psora, either Sycosis or Syphillis or both miasms is/are combined in every man.

One should not be under the impression,

- That **Sulphur, Thuja and Mercurius** alone could antidote **Psoric, Sycotic and Syphilitic** miasms respectively in all cases – **except** the indicated miasmic remedy *as per the theory of "Similia Similibus Curantor" (of Dr. Hahnemann) i.e.* **"symptom-remedy similarity"**.
- Chronic nature of **Digestive Complaint**, have base of **Miasm/s background**, for selection of remedy – – go through the list refered in the **following and pages.**

SELECTION OF REMEDY IN CASE OF ACUTE/CHRONIC AILMENTS

ACUTE AILMENTS

Symptoms continue for a very short period and **come and go in a flash.** When there is a relief the remedy should be **stopped.**

CHRONIC COMPLAINTS:

Repeat from to time, i.e. monthly/quarterly/half-yearly with similar symptoms. Hence the remedies selected to be used starting **generally from 30 potency to 1M** potency depending upon relief. Where there is no relief, the case should be studied once again, go through the present symptoms so as to select a complimentary remedy for the one initially selected **or** when there is **complete change in symptoms** is observed **new remedy** covering the present symptoms to be given.

ANTI – PSORIC, SYCOTIC, AND SYPHILLITIC REMEDIES

Marked with one/or two stars are powerful

ANTI-PSORIC REMEDIES		
Abrotanum	Cistus Canandensis	Muriatic Acid
Acetic Acid	Clematis	Nat.Ars.*
Agaricus Musc	Coccus Cacti	Nat.Carb*
Aloes	Conium *	Nat. Mur**
Alumina*	Crotalus*	Nat.Sulf*
Ambra Grasea	Croton Tig	Nitric Acid*
Ammonium Carb	Cup. Met.	Petroulen
Anacardium*	Digitalis	Phosphorus*
Antimonium Crud	Dulcamara	Phosphoric Acid
Apis Mel*	Ferr.Met.	Platinum

Arg. Met	Ferr.Phos.	Plumbum Met
Ars. Iod.**	Hepar Sulf**	Sarsparilla
Aurum Met*	Iodine**	Secale
Aurum Mur*	Kali Carb*	Selenium*
Baryta Carb*	Kali Iod*	Sepia**
Belladonna	Kali Sulf	Silicea**
Benzoic Acid	Kali Phos	Stanum
Borax	Lac Can*	Staphisgria*
Bufo*	Lachesis**	Sulph.Acid
Carbo Animalis*	Mag.Mur	Tuberculinum**
Carbo Veg*	Manganum	Zincum*
Capsicum*	Mezerium	
ANTI SYCOTIC REMEDIES		
Arg. Met	Kali Iod	Phos.Acid
Arg.Nit	Lycopodium*	Psorinum**
Ars. Alb **	Mag. Carb	Pulsatilla*
Ars. Iod**	Mag. Mur	Pyrogen*
Benz. Acid	Mag. Phos	Sepia**
Berberies Vul	Mezerium**	Sarsparilla
Calc. Ars*	Muriatic Acid	Silicea**
Causticum*	Nat. Ars*	Staphisgria*
Dulcamara	Nat.Carb*	Thuja*
Fluoric Acid	Nat.Mur**	Tuberculinum**
Iodine**	Nat.Sulph	Zincum*
Kali Carb*	Nitric Acid*	
Kali Bich	Phosphorus*	

Remedy covering miasm, more than one miasm, remedy covering in all the three miasms or one or two miasms... Covering in all three miasms, generally happens in the cases of **CANCER/TUBERCULOSIS**

ANTI-SYPHILITIC REMEDIES		ANTI-PSORIC, & SYCOTIC SYPHILLITIC REMEDIES
Ars.Alb.	Lycopodium*	Ars.Alb.
Ars.Iod	Lachesis**	Ars.Iod
Aur.Met*	Mercurius*	Calc.Ars.
Calc.Ars.*	Nitric Acid*	Fluoric Acid
Fluroric Acid	Phytolacca	Kali-Bich
Hepar Sulf**	Staphisgria*	Kali-iod
Kali-Bich*	Sarsparilla	Lycopodium
Kali-Carb*	Syphillinum*	Nitric Acid
Kli-iod*	Tuberculinum	Sarsparilla
		Tuberculinum

Marked with one/or two stars are powerful –

CHAPTER – 2

EVALUATION OF CASE – AETIOLOGY

Whilst evaluations of a case, hurry is the bar, should observe and listen the patient very closely so as to elicit the cause of ailment, observe on the expressions, restlessness and any differences between the couples, Demise of his/her partner or near one, anxiety, or lack of clarity while submitting the symptoms. The following **do's and dont's are to be observed very strictly while taking up a case.**

DON'T

- Put questions in between
- Put leading questions for which the answer is 'yes' or 'no'
- Put embarrassing questions
- Intervene in the middle
- Forget to enquire the modalities – i.e. how the present symptoms are aggravated < or > ameliorated i.e. Relief (a) Only by worm or cold applications/Hot or cold water bathing irrespective of the season. (b) Seasonal differences, (c) Craving for particular taste i.e sweets, spicy, sour etc. or no particularity.

DO'S

- When correct replies are lacking, suggestions can be made to elicit more and more information.

- Ascertain Desires and aversions – i.e. food, drinks and air etc. along with Food habits of the patient.
- Find out the nature of occupation i.e, with mental strain/ physical exertion.
- Ascertain the details of diseases the parents suffered, so that to confirm whether the present symptoms are having any bearing on *hereditary background.*

AETIOLOGY AND ITS IMPORTANCE WHILE TAKING UP A CASE

In some cases Aetiology (*i.e. route cause*) is entirely responsible for the present ailment of the patient. To elicit this, enquire, how and when the present symptoms have come up.

EXAMPLES OF AETIOLOGY AND REMEDIES

AETIOLOGY	REMEDY
Accident/concussions	Arnica
Drenching or wetting head	Rhus Tox
Head Injury	Natrum sulf
Exposure to sun	Glonine or Natrum carb
Exposure to winter or damp cold air	Hepar Sulf or Rhus tox, depending upon the totality of symptoms
Exposure to cold dry air	Aconite
Suppressed anger/insults	Staphisgria
Loss of kith and kin– his partner	Ignatia
Suppressed anger/insults	Staphisgria
Fractures of Bones	Ruta
Headache due to strain of eyes	Gelsimium

Remedies selected just on the pathological symptoms stated presently by the patient without ascertaining **aetiological reasons** will not give the desired results, except the remedy selected **by chance** also covers the aetiological reasons. **Selection of remedy** without eliciting aetiology is like prescribing a remedy from the catalogue of drugs.

- Number of **aetiological factors** are given in the Materia Medica are noted down in alphabetical order so that it can be an **index** to in due course.
- **Noting is very** important to develop knowledge on the theory of homoeopathy, so as to ensure selection of the correct remedy.

Especially the characteristic symptoms of Homoeo remedies are noted in the book in the beginning and in due course they are recorded automatically. Reading, noting, self-study of one's constitution, peculiar symptoms etc. case-study of kith and kin, friends and colleagues, gives more idea of miasms, discussions with experienced homoeopaths will give much knowledge so as to **aim at constitutional remedy** while dealing with chronic complaints – ultimately for a good prognosis of the case.

Also, going through medical journals, articles subscribed by experienced Doctors irrespective of their pathy, gives a **good knowledge on different ailments** of all age groups, from time to time, so that the way of dealing their treatment with Homoeo remedies becomes more easy.

Study every person you come across with the miasmatic view – For example:

- A man with **inverted pyramid** face (i.e. just like letter 'V') is **Psoric**
- A **pointed nose** with beautiful eyes, and structure with thin lips, & curly hair is **Sycotic**
- A **broad face**, with big ears, dwarf personality with dull head, thumb nose and thick lips or bald **is Syphilitic**

One can get this expertise only by thorough and repeated study of physical symptoms of each patient, gets an idea on the constitution, and on 'get up' of the patient having listed his symptoms, it becomes easy to select the constitutional remedy from the lists given earlier in this Chapter, by applying 'Similia Similibus curantor' i.e. remedy-symptoms similarity, of the Patient.

NOTES ON SELECTION OF A REMEDY

(A) REMEDY SELECTION ON THE BASIS OF MIASM

From the Chapters – 1 and Chapter – 2: The readers could follow right from Brief notes on Homoeopathy, Miasms i.e., Psoric, Sycotic, & Syphilis & on the Evaluation of a case – Aetiology, the method of noting the symptoms matching with the Miasms observed from the patients in the Table Form depicted below:

PSORIC	SYCOTIC	SYPHILLITIC

By above method, one could arrive at, under which miasm the symptoms are Major, Medium, or Normal. It is note worthy that in all cases, **Psoric Miasm is a must** as without **Psora**, no person on earth is affected with other Miasms i.e. Sycotic or Siphilis.

Acquaint more with the Table of Miasmatic remedies given **at the end of CHAPTER –1** One should take into the account *majority of symptoms*, worked out against a particular miasm for **selection of remedy:**

Following conclusions for selection of remedy are generally followed by all Homoeopaths.

Cases where – majority of symptoms **are under Psoric Miasm** – than Syphilis or Sycotic, **Select** remedies covering only under **Psoric Miasm.**

Where – majority of symptoms **are under** Sycotic Miasm than Syphilis – **Select** remedies covering **Sycotic Miasm**

When – majority of symptoms **are under** Syphilis Miasm than Sycotic Miasm – **Select** remedies covering **Syphilis Miasm**

At times there may be certain cases when – prominent symptoms/ characteristic symptoms of *all the three miasms,* select remedy *equally* covering all the miasms. *Such instances may arise in case of Cancer, Tuberculosis etc. where there will be symptoms of all the three miasms*

Remedy selection by Repertisation

WHAT IS A REPERTARY?

A repertory is like a dictionary of symptoms arranged systematically from top to bottom of the body i.e. starting from Mind to the lower limbs in an anatomical order and lastly 'Generalities' i.e. in general how the symptoms are aggravated (<) or ameliorated (>) during seasons, timings etc. with each section of the body. The order of aggravation (<) or amelioration (>) of symptoms are given starting from morning to night and with timings wherever necessary.

Grading and Marks of Remedies in the Repertory as under:

Grading: The remedies mentioned in **CAPITALS** are *said to be* **First Grade,** those are in *italics,* **Second grade** & in ordinary type are **Third Grade.**

Marks: at **3** – for **1**st **grade: 2** – **2**nd **grade:** and **1 mark** to **3**rd **grade** remedies respectively allotted are noted after repertisation.

Finally the marks obtained against each remedy **commonly indicated** against the symptoms are totalled. The remedy/ies came out with maximum marks is generally the similimum of the case, **subject to the following norms:**

Just because a certain remedy/ies scored maximum marks, it need not be considered *as the indicated remedy,* when *the mental, peculiar and concomitant symptoms and modalities of the case* are not covered.

On the other hand, Remedies though scored *less marks after repertisation,* if they are covering mental, peculiar and concomitant symptoms and modalities it will be the remedy – Save covering the common/pathological symptoms of the ailment.

Here it is once again mentioned, that one should **thoroughly study** the common symptoms, **so that,** what *is peculiar/concomitant catergory* could be arrived at **to achieve positive results** in the case.

REFERENCE BOOKS

Lectures on Homoeopathic Philosophy by Dr. R.Kent for further study

Chronic diseases its cause and cure by P.N.Bannerje

Chronic diseases by Dr. Hahnemann

Materia Medica by Kent

Kent's Repertory

CHAPTER - 3

PATHOLOGY AND ITS IMPORTANCE IN HOMOEOPATHY

Hahnemann announced his new principle of system of Medicine (Homoeopathy) over 150 years ago. In his time, pathology was practically an underdeveloped science. Whatever little pathology was taught during those periods was full of conjectures, absurd theories and beliefs. For instance, it was thought that the lump sensation felt in the throat by the hysterical women. Under those circumstances Hahnemann had little or no pathological data to go upon and so his theory of totality of symptoms was logical and sound step. The prescriptions were given on the basis of symptoms, although he did agree to the use of pathological changes as guidelines for theoretical purposes. It was his conception at that time pathology will remain imperfect and incomplete and, therefore, to rely entirely on it for **treatment** would be **unwise**. Another reason for ignoring pathology was that there was no experimental proof of the remedies used.

During the last 150 years, there have been tremendous advances in all the medical sciences including medicine, pathology and bacteriology which have totally revolutionized the whole concept of medical sciences. While symptomatology is the real science of therapeutics, yet pathology forms a very important part of symptology by itself. For example, the condition of indigestion, a pathological condition of the stomach, liver or bowel suggest a certain group of remedies as they have effect especially on those organs and thus a great field of materia medica is corner fenced off. In this manner pathology becomes a part of symptomatology.

Pathology helps in individualizing the cases and finding out the remedies according to the organs or system involved. For example — cases of mastoiditis often respond to Capsicum, cancers to Cadmium compounds, splenomegaly to Ceanothus, uterine fibroids to Aurum Mur.Nat and warts to Thuja. Certain drugs show affinity for certain locations, e.g. Sulphur effects lower left lobe of lungs, Kali Carb, Lycopodium, Phosphorous effects right lobe. In the absence of other symptoms, pathological changes may be sure guide in the treatment; say in cases of warts, ulcer etc. So in this way knowledge of pathology helps in selecting the remedy.

Dr. Boger stresses the value of pathological generals as opposed to the diagnostic pathology. He feels that these are the pathological conditions which become characteristic of the patients and affect him in many parts – **Example**, warts, naevi, keloids, polypi, fibroids, tumours, corns etc. – tend to show the constitutional tendency of the person and are, therefore, valuable generals. It is now necessary that we should not be satisfied with mere symptoms, matching them on clinical level, but should go further by correlative studies and clinical observations and try to fit the drug based on the pathological condition.

In Dr. B.K. Sircar's words the knowledge of physiology and pathology is a must for every homoeopath as the homoeopathic approach is based on the idea that similar beginnings lead to similar endings. We are not able to match our remedies to the endings of the diseases e.g. pathology and so we match the beginnings of diseases through characteristic symptoms and on the hypothesis that thereby the ending must also match. However, we must appreciate that this may not always be so and must be able to match the disease and the drug pictures both in their beginnings and endings, e.g. both symptomatically and at the end Pathologically. Otherwise in this age when pathology has so well developed and many disease processes present themselves only through their pathological symptoms, we shall be left behind with our imperfect methods and instruments of cure.

Pathology helps in giving the diagnosis, management of the case including dietary regime and prognosis of a case. Such as a case of diphtheria, it is necessary for a homoeopath to go at once for the pathological findings and give a correct diagnosis. If he is not able to do so, it will be impossible for him to handle the case.

Pathology is an indispensable auxiliary branch to the study of the subject of therapeutics. It is helpful in enabling the physician to group the symptoms of a case in a more rational way. Pathology acts not only as a guide in therapeutics but also acts as an instrument which he uses in studying the phenomenon which are the respectively the subject and agents of his therapeutic operation. When we take the symptomatology as a picture of totality of the symptoms, external and internal causes, and course of the disease, then pathology is indispensable to therapeutics.

In summary, the knowledge of the pathology is necessary for selection of correct similimum.

CHAPTER – 4

TWELVE TISSUE REMEDIES (BIO-CHEMIC SALTS) BASIC PRINCIPLES

The foundation of Bio-chemistry was laid more than a Century ago, when Rudolph Virchow, one of the foremost scientists of the day, discovered that the human body is composed of an enormous number of tiny, living cells, each one made up of infinitesimal but perfectly in a balanced quantity of three classes of material – **Water, Organic Substances and Inorganic Substances.**

Organic matter constitutes sugar, albuminous and fatty substances which make up the greater portion of the body. The salts constitute inorganic components. These inorganic substances are present in very much smaller quantities, and are vital elements, active workers which utilize the organic substances in building the millions of cells of which the body is composed.

Millions of cells of the body will be constantly breaking down and new ones are rapidly built up with the help of necessary materials, supplied from blood stream. In the absence of inorganic elements, the rebuilding process of cells cannot proceed in a normal orderly manner. Disturbance of the bodily rhythm gives rise to what is called 'DISEASE' in one of its many and varied forms. **Disease means lack of ease and indicates a disturbance of the bodily rhythm.**

A shortage or deficiency of one or several of these vital mineral substances (inorganic substances) may arise from a variety of causes: injuries, self-poisoning and obscure influences which in many instances science has not yet been able to explain. The invisible natural forces within us are the most effective guardians of our health. However, even these great natural forces are unable to keep the complicated human structure, in good working order, if the blood does not contain the materials required for the building of new healthy cells.

INORGANIC CONSTITUENTS OF CELLS

The principal inorganic materials of nerve-cells are Magnesia Phos, Kali Phos, Natrum and Ferrum. Muscle-Cells contain the same, with the addition of Kali Mur. Connective tissue-cells have for their specific substance Silicea, while that the elastic tissue-cells is probably Calcarea Flour. In bone-cells we have Calcarea Fluor, and Magnesia Phos and a large proportion of Calcarea Phos, and Calc. Phos in small quantities in the cells of muscle, nerve, brain and connective tissues. Natrum Mur (common salt) is contained in the cartilages, mucous cells, and in the fluid parts of the body in solid form.

These inorganic substances are found in the tissues of the body in minute molecular form, say equaling to 6x level, and when these salts are deficient in the tissues, gaps are formed in molecular level. Therefore, to fill in these gaps, the salts are required to be given in the same form (molecular form) probably in 6x potency (decimal potency) for giving desired results towards cure. Thus molecule of tissue salt chosen for treatment replaces the gaps caused in the tissues of the body and eliminate the symptoms caused due to its deficiency. Keeping these aspects, Dr. Scheussler has found out the concept of Bio-chemistry, and prepared the following 12 tissue remedies, and was successful in getting results for fighting with the disease caused due to their deficiency in the tissues of the body.

There are 12 tissue salts, which are in use, and their indications are given against them. They are generally used in 6x potency. –Dosage 4 tablets each time at 8AM, 12AM, 4PM and 8PM (four times a day) say for a period of 15 days, month to 6 months with interval of 5 days in between for every course depending on relief. If relief is found in all cases further doses to be stopped.

Sl No.	Salt	Bio-chemical action of salt – its deficiency – their indications
01	Calc. Fl.	This salt gives to the tissues the quality of elasticity. It combines with organic substances, albumin, to form organic tissue and is found in the walls of the blood vessels, muscular tissues, connective tissue,and the surface of bones and in the enamel of teeth. A deficiency of Calcarea Flour results in a loss of elasticity and consequent relaxed condition – e.g. relaxed condition of veins and arteries, piles, sluggish circulation, a tendency to cracks in the skin, notably in the palms of the hands, and between the toes. Due to its deficiency the elasticity in the muscular tissue and supporting membranes become impaired,resulting in muscular weakness, bearing down pains etc. – condition sare relieved by massage and warmth.
02	Calc. Phos	Calc. Phos is the tissue salt concerned with nutrition. It combines with albumin and is indicated when there are albuminous discharges. It promotes healthy cellular activity and restores tone to weakend organs and tissues. Bone and teeth troubles and thus becomes important remedy for children – useful for normal growth. A good remedy for rickets – for joining the fractures in bones.
03	Calc Sulph	Calc.Sulph is a blood purifier and healer. It supplements the action of Kali-mur in the treatment of catarrh acne, etc. and it should always be given when 'pimples' occur in adolescence. It checks the weakening drain of pus due to which suppuration is continued too long, e.g. abscesses and wounds which would not heal readily and tend to become septic. A good medicine to be thought of for sinusitis – symptoms are generally worse after getting wet and in a warm dry atmosphere.

Continued...

Sl No.	Salt	Bio-chemical action of salt – its deficiency – their indications
04	Ferr.phos	It is the pre-eminent bio-chemic first aid remedy. It is the oxygen carrier – congestive inflammatory pains, high temperature –quickened pulse, all for more oxygen, and it is Ferr. Phos that is the medium through which oxygen is taken up by the blood stream and carried to the affected area and hence a good remedy for all firststage inflammations anywhere. Painful blood boils – Bleeding from wounds, cuts and abrasions can be controlled with a little powder of Ferr. Phos applied direct to the injured parts, externally. For this purpose crush few tablets and prepare lotion and apply externally.
05	Kali. Mur	Kali-Mur is the remedy for sluggish conditions. It combines with the organic substances, fibrin. The discharges are white fibrinous. With Calc. Sulph it can be used for cleansing and purifying the blood. In alternation with Ferr. Phos it is very effective remedy for treatment of inflammatory diseases, particularly those affecting respiration, coughs, colds, sore throats, tonslitis, bronchitis etc. A good remedy in children for measles, chicken pox and mumps – painful boils. Inflammation with much pain.
06	Kali. Phos	It is a nerve nutrient. Ailments of a truly nervous character.School children often need this tissue salts; it helps to maintain a happy contented disposition and sharpens mental faculties. In these cases the early symptoms are fretfulness, ill-humored. bashfulness, timidity, laziness. A good remedy for nervous headaches, nervous dyspepsia (painful digestion), sleeplessness, depression; In one word it is a good nerve and brain tonic
07	Kali. Sulph	It works in conjunction with Ferr. Phos as an oxygen – carrier. Desires for cool open air – Promotes perspiration in fevers and reduces the fever. A good remedy for dandruff – symptoms are generally worse in the evening, or in a closed stuffy atmosphere, and are better in the fresh air.

Sl No.	Salt	Bio-chemical action of salt – its deficiency – their indications
08	Mag. Phos	It is known as the anti-spasmodic tissue salt. It supplements the action of Kali-phos in nerve disorders. A good remedy for cramps, spasmodic pains. Muscular pains, nerve pains, such as neuralgia, neuritis, sciatica and headaches accompanied by shooting darting stabs of pain. Painful menstruation. Pains better by warm applications. To get good results during pain mix 6 or 10 tables of 6x potency in warm water and give it in tea-spoonful doses at hourly intervals.
09	Nat. Phos	Acid neutralizing tissue remedy and neutralize the acid conditions. It is the principal remedy for the wide group of ailments from the joints resulting in stiffness and swelling and other painful rheumatic symptoms. Acid dyspepsia – Sleeplessness caused by indigestion can be relieved. A good remedy for worm symptoms in children
10	Nat. Mur	It attracts water to equally distribute to the tissues. Excessive moisture or excessive dryness are the indications for this remedy. Headaches due to constipation – A good remedy for constipation in conjunction with Calc. Phos for children – Water discharge from nose – Is a good remedy for cold symptoms with running of nose – this is to be thought of in summer as much salt is lost due to sweating.
11	Nat. Sulph	It regulates the density of the intercellular fluids (fluids which bath the tissue cells) by eliminating excess water. It attracts the water from the tissues to eliminate – It is a liver tonic and ensure its healthy functioning – A good remedy for diabetes Mellitus or Insipidus. This is to be thought of in respiratory troubles in damp – weather, so think of in Asthma. Wind in the intestines – Salt to be thought in Jaundice.

Continued...

Sl No.	Salt	Bio-chemical action of salt – its deficiency – their indications
12	Silicea	It is a third salt to be thought of as a cleanser and eliminator of toxins of the tissues. It will help in eliminating the pus formed in various parts of the body tissues. Its deficiency in tissues causes pus formations. It breaks up the long standing abscesses and cleans there. It is a scavenger of the body in conjunction with Kali. Mur. To be thought of whenever pus formations are there – Good remedy in sinusitis with pus in the ears or in tonsillitis.

WHETHER BIO-CHEMIC SALTS CAN BE USED IN COMBINATIONS?

Bio-chemic salts can be used in combination of one or two so as to cover the totality of the symptoms caused due to their deficiencies. Such combinations are given below and available in all the Homoeo Medical stores. The numbers are similarly denoted by different suppliers of these combinations, though the patent name of the combination may differ i.e. **BYCO, BIO-GEN or BIO-PLAST** etc. Dosage 4 tablets each time at 8AM, 12AM, 4PM and 8PM (four times a day) say for a period of 15 days, month to 6 months with interval of 5 days in between for every course depending on relief. If relief is found in all cases stop the medicine.

Sl. No.	Nature of complaint	Combination
01	Anaemia	CP 3x, FP 3x, NM 6x, and KP 3x
02	Asthma	KP 3x, MP 3x, NM 6x, NS 3x
03	Colic	KP 3x, MP 3x, CP 3x, NS 6x, FP 3X
04	Constipation	CP 3x, CF 3x, KM 3x, NM 3x, Sil. 6x
05	Coryza	FP 3x, KM 3x, KS 3X, 3x, NM 6x
06	Cough, Cold & Catarrah	FP 3x, KM 3x, MP 3x, NM 6x, NS 6x
07	Diabetes	CP 3x, FP 3x, KP 3x, NP 3x, NS 6x
09	Dysentery	FP 3x, KM 3x, KP 3x, MP 3x
10	Enlarged Tonsils	CP 3x, FP 3x, KM 3x,
11	Fever	FP 3x, KM 3x, KS 3X, NM 3x, NS 3x,

12	Headache	FP 3x, KP 3x, MP 3x, NM 3x
13	Leucorrhoea	CS 3X, CP 3x, KP 3x, KS 3x, NM 3x
15	Menstrual disorders	CP 3x, FP 3x, KP36x, KS 3x, MP 6x
16	Nervous Exhaustion	CP3x, FP 3x, KP 6x, MP 3x, NM 3x
17	Piles	CF 3x, FP 3x, CP 3x, KM 6x
18	Pyorrhea	CF 3x, CS 3x, Sil.6x
19	Rheumatism	CP 3x, FP 3x, KS 3x, MP 3x, NS 6x
20	Skin diseases	CF 6x, CS 6x, KS 3x, NM 6x, NS 6x
21	Teething trouble	CP 3x, FP 3x
22	Scrofula	CP 3x, FP 3x, KM 36x, Sil. 6x
23	Toothache	CF 3x, FP 3x, KP 3x,KM 3x, Sil. 6x
24	Tonic Brain & Nerves	CP 3x, FP 3x, KP 3x, MP 3x, NP 3x
25	Acidity, Flatulence – Indigestion	NP 3x, NS 6x, Sil.12x
26	Easy parturition	CP 3x, CF 3x, KP 3x, MP 3x
27	Lack of vitality	CP 6x, KP 3x, NS 6x
28	General Tonic	All the twelve tissue salts IN 6X

Abreviations addressed

CF – Calcarea Fluor	KM – Kali Mur	NM – Natrum Mur
CP – Calcarea Phos	KP – Kali Phos	NP – Natrum Phos
CS – Calcarea Sulph	KS – Kali Sulph	NS – Natrum Sulph
FP – Ferrum Phos	MP – Magnesia Phos	Sil – Silicea

When the above **combinations do not cover** the totality of the symptoms of the case, pick up the suitable salts – (in 6x potency) so as to prepare a Bio-combination to suit the present symptoms. (At 2 pinches of powder of the mix – per dose.)

WHEN TO USE BIO-SALTS?

Used directly in the cases of complaints of tissue degenerations, or for boosting due to their deficiency the patient kept purely on Bio-salts.

Where Homoeopathic treatment is on, initially, two doses of the **Homoeopathy remedy** selected is given. Thereafter it will be stopped for about 15 days. During 15 days interval, the indicated bio-chemic salt or the combination of salts could be used 3 times per day as under – depending upon the relief obtained after using the indicated Homoeopathy remedy i.e where there is complete relief **bio-chemic need not be used.**

The need for Bio –chemic remedy generally do not occur in Acute complaints except in Chronic cases.

In **Chronic complaints,** the **bio-chemic salts** are prescribed, only **during the interval** after giving Homoeopathy remedy, depending upon the prognosis.

Timings of Bio-salts in all cases are preferably @ **8AM, 2PM and 8PM** – May not Scrupulously be followed but 3 doses are to be given with **4 hours** gap between each dose.

Bio-chemic remedies – single/combinations? – In Acute Complaints the remedies of single salt to be given. In Chronic cases combination of salts only are to be prescribed. **Examples are as under:**

Case – 1: (Single salt – Nat Phos)

Peptic Ulcer – remedy – **Kali-bich** – Two doses of Kali-bich are given, with a gap of 15 days – **Nat Phos 6x** – @ **3 doses,** for complementing the action of

Kali-bich, so as to help in healing of ulcerated tissue in the stomach or duodenum as the case may be.

Case – 2: (Combination – 12)

Chronic headache, (**Remedy – Spigelia**) Two doses of the remedy are given – During 15 days gap, Bio combination No.12 is given at **3 doses as indicated above** (Combination No.12 is indicated for Headache)

REFERENCE BOOKS

Twelve Tissue Remedies of "By Schussler – William Boericke & Willis A.Dewey

CHAPTER – 5

ANATOMY & PHYSIOLOGY OF DIGESTIVE TRACT

A Physician should possess the importance right from the Anatomy and Physiology and on Ailments of Digestive Tract in brief and pathological importance is asserted **so as to pin point actual cause for the present ailment** of patients approaching to Homoeopath – as a technician to repair the unit entrusted to him for repair.

The **Gastrointestinal System** is responsible for breakdown & absorption of various foods, liquids needed to sustain life. Many different organs have essential roles in the digestion of food, from the mechanical disrupting by the teeth to the creation of bile (an emulsifier) by the liver. Bile production of liver plays an important role in digestion, from being stored and concentrated in the gallbladder during fasting stages to being discharged to the small intestine.

In order to understand the interactions of the different components we shall follow the food on its **journey** through the human body. During digestion, two main processes occur at the same time namely:

- **Mechanical Digestion:** Larger pieces of food get broken down into smaller pieces while being prepared for chemical digestion. Mechanical digestion starts in mouth and continues into the stomach.
- **Chemical Digestion:** Starts in mouth and continues into the intestines. Several different enzymes break down

macromolecules into smaller molecules that can be absorbed. The GI tract starts with the mouth and proceeds to the esophagus, stomach, small intestine (duodenum, jejunum, ileum), and then to the large intestine (colon), rectum, and terminates at the anus.

You could probably say the human body is just like a big donut. The GI tract is the donut hole. We will also be discussing the pancreas and liver, and accessory organs of the gastrointestinal system that contribute materials to the small intestine.

Layers of GI Tract: The GI tract is composed of four layers also known as **Tunics**. Each layer has different tissues and functions. From the inside out they are called: **Mucosa, Sub-mucosa, Muscularis, and Serosa.**

Mucosa: The mucosa is the absorptive and secretory layer. It is composed of simple epithelium cells and a thin connective tissue. There are specialized goblet cells that secrete mucus throughout the GI tract located within the mucosa. On the mucosa layer there are **Villi and Micro Villi.**

Sub-mucosa: The sub mucosa is relatively thick, highly vascular, and serves the mucosa. The absorbed elements that pass through the mucosa are picked up from blood vessels of the sub mucosa. The sub mucosa also has glands and nerve plexuses.

Muscularis: The muscularis is responsible for segmental contractions and peristaltic movement in the GI tract. The muscularis is composed of two layers of **muscle: an inner circular and outer longitudinal** layer of smooth muscle. These muscles cause food to move and churn with digestive enzymes down the **GI tract.**

Serosa: The last layer is a protective layer. It is composed of avascular connective tissue and simple squamous epithelium. It secretes lubricating serous fluid. This is the visible layer on the outside of the organs.

ACCESSORY ORGANS

1. Salivary glands: Parotid gland, submandibular gland, sublingual gland Exocrine gland that produces saliva which begins the process of digestion with amylase.

2. Tongue: Manipulates food for chewing/swallowing – Main taste organ, covered in taste buds.

3. Teeth: For chewing food up

4. Liver: Produces and excretes bile required for emulsifying fats. Some of the bile drains directly into the duodenum and some is stored in the gall bladder. Helps metabolize proteins, lipids, and carbohydrates. – – Urea, chief end product of mammalian metabolism, is formed in liver from amino acids and compounds of ammonia. – – – Breaks down insulin and other hormones. – – – Produces coagulation factors.

5. Gallbladder: Bile storage.

6. Pancreas

- Exocrine functions: Digestive enzyme secretion.
- Stores zymogens (inactive enzymes) that will be activated by the brush border membrane in the small intestine when a person eats protein (amino acids).
- Trypsinogen – Trypsin: digests protein.
- Chymotypsinogen – Chymotrypsin: digests proteins.
- Carboxypeptidase's: digests proteins.
- Lipase-lipid: digests fats.
- Amylase: digests carbohydrates.
- Endocrine functions: Hormone secretion.

Somatostatin: Inhibits the function of insulin. Produce if the body is getting too much glucose.

Glucagons: Stimulates the stored glycogen in the liver to convert to glucose. Produced if the body does not have enough glucose.

Insulin: made in the beta cells of the Islets of Langerhans of the pancreas. Insulin is a hormone that regulates blood glucose.

7. Vermiform appendix

There are a few theories on what the appendix does.

- Vestigal organ
- Immune function
- Helps maintain gut flora

First step in the digestive system can actually begin before the food is even in the mouth. The smell or sight of food to eat, start salivation in anticipation of eating, thus beginning the digestive process.

Food is the body's source of fuel. Nutrients in food give the body's cells the energy they need to operate. Before food can be used it has to be broken down into tiny little pieces so that it can be absorbed and used by the body. In humans, proteins need to be broken down into amino acids, starches into sugars, and fats into fatty acids and glycerol.

The digestive system is made up by the alimentary canal, or the digestive tract, and other abdominal organs that play a part in digestion such as the liver and the pancreas. The alimentary canal is the long tube of organs that runs from the mouth (where the food enters) to the anus (where indigestible waste leaves). The organs in the alimentary canal include the mouth (for mastication), esophagus, stomach and the intestines. The average adult digestive tract is about thirty feet (30') long. While in the digestive tract the food is really passing *through* the body rather than being in the body. The smooth muscles of the tubular digestive organs move the food efficiently along as it is broken down into absorbable atoms and molecules. During absorption, the nutrients that come from food (such as proteins, fats, carbohydrates, vitamins, and minerals) pass through the wall of the small intestine and into the bloodstream and lymph. In this way nutrients can be distributed throughout the rest of the body. In the large intestine there is reabsorption of water and absorption of some minerals as feaces are formed. The parts of the food that the body passes out through the anus is known as feaces.

MASTICATION

Digestion begins in the mouth. A brain reflex triggers the flow of saliva when we see or even think about food. Saliva moistens the food while the teeth chew it up and make it easier to swallow. Amylase, which is the digestive enzyme found in saliva, starts to break down starch into simpler sugars before the food even leaves the mouth. The nervous pathway involved in salivary excretion requires stimulation of receptors in the mouth, sensory impulses to the brain stem, and parasympathetic impulses to salivary glands.

Swallowing food happens when the muscles in the tongue and mouth move the food into **pharynx**. The pharynx, which is the passage way for food and air, is about five inches (5") long. A small flap of skin called the epiglotitis closes over the pharynx to prevent food from entering the trachea and thus choking. For swallowing to happen correctly a combination of 25 muscles must all work together at the same time.

Salivary glands produce an estimated Three liters of saliva per day

Enzyme	Produced In	Site of Release	pH Level
Carbohydrate Digestion			
Salivary amylase	Salivary glands	Mouth	Neutral
Pancreatic amylase	Pancreas	Small intestine	Basic
Maltase	Small intestine	Small intestine	Basic

Continued...

Protein Digestion			
Pepsin	Gastric glands	Stomach	Acidic
Trypsin	Pancreas	Small intestine	Basic
Peptidases	Small intestine	Small intestine	Basic
Nucleic Acid Digestion			
Nuclease	Pancreas	Small intestine	Basic
Nucleosidases	Pancreas	Small intestine	Basic
Fat Digestion			
Lipase	Pancreas	Small intestine	Basic

MOUTH & ITS PHYSIOLOGY

The **Esophagus** (also spelled oesophagus/esophagus) or gullet is the muscular tube in vertebrates through which ingested food passes from the throat to the stomach. The esophagus is continuous with the laryngeal part of the pharynx at the level of the C6 vertebra. It connects the pharynx, which is the body cavity that is common to both the digestive and respiratory systems behind the mouth, with the stomach, where the second stage of digestion is initiated (the first stage is in the mouth with teeth and tongue masticating food and mixing it with saliva).

After passing through the throat, the food moves into the esophagus and is pushed down into the stomach by the process of *peristalsis* (involuntary wavelike muscle contractions along the G.I. tract). At the end of the esophagus there is a **sphincter** that allows food into the stomach then closes back up so the food cannot travel back up into the esophagus.

Esophagus – Histology The esophagus is lined **with** mucus membranes, and uses *peristaltic action* to move swallowed food down to the stomach. The esophagus is lined by a *stratified squamous epithelium*, which is rapidly turned over, and serves a protective effect due to the high volume transit of food, saliva, and mucus into the stomach. The *lamina propria* of the esophagus is sparse. The mucus secreting glands are located in the sub mucosa, and are connective structures called *papillae*.

The muscular is propria of the esophagus consists of *striated muscle* in the upper third (superior) part of the esophagus. The middle third consists of a combination of *smooth muscle* and striated muscle, and the bottom (inferior) third is only smooth muscle. The distal end of the esophagus is slightly narrowed because of the thickened circular muscles. **This part of the esophagus is called the lower esophageal sphincter. This aids in keeping food down and not being regurgitated. The esophagus has a rich** *lymphatic* drainage as well.

STOMACH & ITS PHYSIOLOGY

The Stomach is a thick walled organ that lies between the esophagus and the first part of the small intestine (the duodenum). It is on the left side of the abdominal cavity, the fundus of the stomach lying against the diaphragm. Lying beneath the stomach is the pancreas. The greater omentum hangs from the greater curvature. A mucous membrane lines the stomach which contains glands (with *chief cells*) that secrete gastric juices, up to three quarts of this digestive fluid is produced daily. The gastric glands begin secreting before food enters the stomach due to the parasympathetic impulses of the *vagus nerve*, making the stomach also a storage vat for that acid.

The secretion of gastric juices occurs in three phases: *Cephalic, Gastric, and Intestinal.* The cephalic phase is activated by the smell and taste of food and swallowing. The gastric phase is activated by the chemical effects of food and the distension of the stomach. The intestinal phase blocks the effect of the cephalic and gastric phases. Gastric juice also contains an enzyme named **pepsin**, which digests proteins, hydrochloric acid and mucus. Hydrochloric acid causes the stomach to maintain a pH of about 2, which helps to kill off bacteria that comes into the digestive system via food.

The gastric juice is highly acidic with a pH of 1–3. It may cause or compound damage to the stomach wall or its layer of mucus, causing a peptic ulcer. On the inside of the stomach there are folds of skin call the gastric rugae. Gastric rugae make the stomach very extendable, especially after a very big meal.

The stomach is divided into four sections, each of which has different cells and functions. The sections are: (1) Cardiac region, where the contents of the esophagus empty into the stomach, (2) Fundus, formed by the upper curvature of the organ, (3) Body, the main central region, and (4) Pylorus or atrium, the lower section of the organ that facilitates emptying the contents into the small intestine. Two smooth muscle valves, or sphincters, keep the contents of the stomach contained. They are the: (1) Cardiac or esophageal sphincter, dividing the tract above, and (2) Pyloric sphincter, dividing the stomach from the small intestine.

After receiving the **bolus** (chewed food) the process of peristalsis is started; mixed and churned with gastric juices the bolus is transformed into a semi-liquid substance called **chyme**. Stomach muscles mix up the food with enzymes and acids to make smaller digestible pieces. The pyloric sphincter, a walnut shaped muscular tube at the stomach outlet, keeps chyme in the stomach until it reaches the right consistency to pass into small intestine. The food leaves stomach in small squirts rather than all at once.

Water, alcohol, salt, and simple sugars can be absorbed directly through stomach wall. However, most substances in our food need a little more digestion and must travel into intestines before they can be absorbed. *When the stomach is empty it is about the size of one fifth of a cup of fluid. When stretched and expanded, it can hold up to eight cups of food after a big meal.*

Gastric Glands:There are many different gastric glands and they secret many different chemicals. Parietal cells secrete hydrochloric acid and intrinsic factor; chief cells secrete pepsinogen; goblet cells secrete mucus; argentaffin cells secrete serotonin and histamine; and G cells secrete the hormone gastrin.

VESSELS AND NERVES

Arteries: Arteries supplying the stomach are the left gastric, right gastric and right gastro-epiploic branches of the hepatic, left gastro-epiploic and short gastric branches of the lineal. They supply the muscular coat, ramify in the sub mucous coat, and are finally distributed to the mucous membrane.

Capillaries: The arteries break up at the base of the gastric tubules into a plexus of fine capillaries, which run upward between the tubules, anatomizing with each other, and ending in a plexus of larger capillaries, which surround the mouths of the tubes, and also form hexagonal meshes around the ducts.

Veins: From these the veins arise, and pursue a straight course downward, between the tubules, to the sub mucous tissue; they end either in the lineal and superior mesenteric veins, or directly in the portal vein.

Lymphatics: The lymphatics are numerous: They consist of a superficial and a deep set, and pass to the lymph glands found along the two curvatures of the organ.

NERVES IN THE LOWER ABDOMEN

The nerves are the terminal branches of right and left urethra and other parts, the former being distributed upon the back, and the latter upon the front part of the organ. A great number of branches from the celiac plexus of the sympathetic are also distributed to it. Nerve plexuses are found in the sub mucous coat and muscular coat as in the intestine. From these plexuses fibrils are distributed to the muscular tissue & the mucous membrane.

DISORDERS OF THE STOMACH

Disorders of the stomach are common. There can be many different causes with a variety of symptoms. The strength of the inner lining of the stomach needs a careful balance of acid and mucus. If there is not enough mucus in the stomach, ulcers, abdominal pain, indigestion, heartburn, nausea and vomiting could all be caused by the extra acid. Erosions, ulcers, and tumours can cause bleeding. When blood is in the stomach it starts the digestive process and turns black. When this happens, the person can have black stool or vomit. Some ulcers can bleed very slowly so the person won't recognize the loss of blood. Over time, the iron in your body will run out, which in turn, will cause anemia.

There is no known diet to prevent getting ulcers.

A balanced, healthy diet is always recommended. Smoking can also be a cause of problems in the stomach. *Tobacco increases acid production and damages the lining of the stomach*. It is not a proven fact that stress alone can cause an ulcer.

HISTOLOGY OF THE HUMAN STOMACH

Like the other parts of the gastrointestinal tract, the stomach walls are made of a number of layers. From inside to the outside, the first main layer is the mucosa. This consists of an epithelium, the lamina propria underneath, and a thin bit of smooth muscle called the *muscularis mucosa*.

Sub mucosa lies under this and consists of fibrous connective tissue, separating the mucosa from the next layer, the *muscularis* **external**. The muscularis in the stomach differs from that of other GI organs in that it has three layers of muscle instead of two. Under these muscle layers is the adventitia, layers of connective tissue continuous with the omenta.

The epithelium of the stomach forms deep pits, called fundic or oxyntic glands. Different types of cells are at different locations down the pits. The cells at the base of these pits are chief cells, responsible for production of pepsinogen, an inactive precursor of pepsin, which degrades proteins. The secretion of pepsinogen prevents self-digestion of the stomach cells.

Further up the pits, parietal cells produce gastric acid and a vital substance, intrinsic factor. The function of gastric acid is two-fold (1) it kills most of the bacteria in food, stimulates hunger, and activates pepsinogen into pepsin, and (2) denatures the complex protein molecule as a precursor to protein digestion through enzyme action in the stomach and small intestines. Near the top of the pits, closest to the contents of the stomach, there are mucous-producing cells called goblet cells that help protect the stomach from self-digestion.

The **muscularis externa** is made up of three layers of smooth muscle. The innermost layer is obliquely-oriented: this is not seen in other parts of the digestive system: this layer is responsible for creating the motion that churns and physically breaks down the food. The next layers are the square and then the longitudinal, which are present as in other parts of the GI tract. The pyloric antrum which has thicker skin cells in its walls and performs more forceful contractions than the fundus. The pylorus is surrounded by a thick circular muscular wall which is normally tonically constricted forming a functional (if not anatomically discrete) pyloric sphincter, which controls the movement of chyme.

Control of secretion and motility: The movement and the flow of chemicals into the stomach are controlled by both the nervous system and by the various digestive system hormones. The hormone **gastrin** causes an increase in the secretion of HCL, pepsinogen and intrinsic factor from parietal cells in the stomach. It also causes increased motility in the stomach.

Gastrin is released by G-cells into the stomach. It is inhibited by pH normally less than 4 (high acid), as well as the hormone somatostatin.

Cholecystokinin (CCK) has most effect on the gall bladder, but it also decreases gastric emptying. In a different and rare manner, secretion, produced in the small intestine, has most effects on the pancreas, but will also diminish acid secretion in the stomach.

Gastric inhibitory peptide (GIP) and enteroglucagon decrease both gastric motility and secretion of pepsin. Other than gastrin, these hormones act to turn off the stomach action. This is in response to food products in the liver and gall bladder, which have not yet been absorbed. The stomach needs only to push food into the small intestine when the intestine is not busy. While the intestine is full and still digesting food, the stomach acts as a storage for food.

The small intestine: – The small intestine is the site where most of the chemical and mechanical digestion is carried out. Tiny projections called **villi** line the small intestine which absorbs digested food into the capillaries. Most of the food absorption takes place in the jejunum and the ileum.

The functions of a small intestine is, the digestion of proteins into peptides and amino acids principally occurs in the stomach but some also occurs in the small intestine. Peptides are degraded into amino acids; lipids (fats) are degraded into fatty acids and glycerol; and carbohydrates are degraded into simple sugars. The three main sections of the small intestine are *duodenum, jejunum and ileum.*

Duodenum: – In anatomy of the digestive system, **duodenum** is a hollow jointed tube connecting stomach to the jejunum. It is the first and shortest part of small intestine. It begins with duodenal bulb and ends at ligament of Treitz. Duodenum is almost entirely retro peritoneal and also where the bile and pancreatic juices enter the intestine.

Jejunum: – *Jejunum* is a part of the small bowel, located between distal end of duodenum and proximal part of ileum. The jejunum and the ileum are suspended by an extensive mesentery giving the bowel great mobility within the abdomen. The inner surface of jejunum, its mucous membrane is covered in projections called villi, which increase the surface area of tissue available to absorb nutrients from the gut contents.

It is different from ileum due to fewer goblet cells and generally lacks Peyer›s patches.

Ileum: – Its function is to absorb vitamin B12 and bile salts. The wall itself is made up of folds, each of which has many tiny finger-like projections known as villi, on its surface. In turn, the epithelial cells which line these villi possess even larger numbers of micro villi. The cells that line the ileum contain protease and carbohydrate enzymes responsible for final stages of protein and carbohydrate digestion. These enzymes are present in the cytoplasm of epithelial cells. The villi contain large numbers of capillaries which take the amino acids and glucose produced by digestion to hepatic portal vein and the liver.

The terminal ileum continues to absorb bile salts, and is also crucial in the absorption of fat-soluble vitamins (Vitamin A, D, E and K). For fat-soluble vitamin absorption to occur, bile acids must be present.

Large Intestine: – Large intestine (colon) extends from the end of ileum to the anus. It is about 5 feet long, being one-fifth of whole extent of intestinal canal. It's caliber is largest at the commencement of the ceacum, and gradually diminishes as far as the rectum, where there is a dilatation of considerable size just above the anal canal. It differs from the small intestine in by the greater caliber, more fixed position, sacculated form, and in possessing certain appendages to its external coat, the appendices epiploicæ. Further, its longitudinal muscular fibers do not form a continuous layer around the gut, but are arranged in three longitudinal bands or tæniæ.

The large intestine is divided into the **ceacum, colon, rectum, and anal canal.** In its course, describes an arch which surrounds the convolutions of the small intestine. It commences in the right iliac region, in a dilated part, the ceacum. It ascends through the right lumbar and hypochondriac regions to the under surface of the liver; here it takes a bend, the right colic flexure, to the left and passes transversely across the abdomen on the confines of the epigastric and umbilical regions, to the left hypochondriac region; it then bends again, the left colic flexure, and descends through the left lumbar and iliac regions to the pelvis, where it forms a bend called the sigmoid flexure; from this it is continued along the posterior wall of the pelvis to the anus.

There are trillions of bacteria, yeasts, and parasites living in intestines, mostly in the colon. Over 400 species of organisms live in the colon. Most of these are very helpful to our health, while the minority are harmful. Helpful organisms *synthesize* vitamins, like *B12*, *biotin*, and *vitamin K*. They break-down toxins and stop proliferation of harmful organisms and stimulate the immune system and produce short chain fatty acids (SCFAs) that are required for the health of colon cells and help to prevent colon cancer. There are many beneficial bacteria but some of the most common and important are *Lactobacilus Acidophilus* and various species of *Bifidobacterium*. These are available as «probiotics» from many sources

Pancreas, Liver, and Gallbladder: – The pancreas, liver, and gallbladder are essential for digestion. The pancreas produces enzymes that helps to digest proteins, fats, and carbohydrates, the liver produces bile that helps the body absorb fat, and the gallbladder stores the bile until it is needed. The enzymes and bile travel through special channels called ducts and into the small intestine where they help break down of the food.

Pancreas: – The **pancreas** is located posterior to the stomach and in close association with the duodenum. In humans, the pancreas is a 6–10 inch elongated organ in the abdomen located retro peritoneal. It is often described as having three regions: a head, body and tail. The pancreatic head abuts the second part of the duodenum while the tail extends towards the spleen. The pancreatic duct runs the length of the pancreas and empties into the second part of duodenum at the ampulla of Vater. The common bile duct commonly joins the pancreatic duct at or near this point.

Pancreas is supplied arterially by the pancreatico-duodenal arteries, themselves branches of the superior mesenteric artery of the hepatic artery (branch of celiac trunk from the abdominal aorta). The superior mesenteric artery provides the inferior pancreatico-duodenal arteries while the gastro-duodenal artery (one of the terminal branches of the hepatic artery) provides the superior pancreatico-duodenal artery. Venous drainage is **via** the pancreatic duodenal veins which end up in the portal vein. The splenicvein passed posterior to the pancreas but is said not drain the pancreas itself. The portal vein is formed by the union of the superior mesenteric vein and splenic vein posterior to the body of the pancreas. In some people (as many as 40%) the inferior mesenteric vein also joins with the splenic vein behind the pancreas, in others it simply joins with the superior mesenteric vein instead.

The function of the pancreas is to produce enzymes that break down all categories of digestible foods (exocrine pancreas) and secrete hormones that affect carbohydrates metabolism (endocrine pancreas).

Exocrine: – The pancreas is composed of pancreatic exocrine cells, whose ducts are arranged in clusters called acini (singular acinus). The cells are filled with secretory granules containing the precursor digestive enzymes (mainly trypsinogen, chymotrypsinogen, pancreatic lipase, and amylase) that are secreted into the lumen of the acinus. These granules are termed zymogen granules (zymogen referring to the inactive precursor enzymes.) It is important to synthesize inactive enzymes in the pancreas to avoid auto degradation, which can lead to pancreatitis.

The pancreas is near the liver, and is the main source of enzymes for digesting fats (lipids) and proteins – the intestinal walls have enzymes that will digest polysaccharides. Pancreatic secretions from ductal cells contain bicarbonate ions and are alkaline in order to neutralize the acidic chyme that the stomach churns out. Control of the exocrine function of the pancreas are via the hormone gastrin, cholecystokinin and secretin, which are hormones secreted by cells in the stomach and duodenum, in response to distension and/or food and which causes secretion of pancreatic juices.

The two major proteases which the pancreas are trypsinogen & chymotrypsinogen. These zymogens are inactivated forms of trypsin and chymotrypsin. Once released in the intestine, the enzyme enterokinase present in the intestinal mucosa activates trypsinogen by cleaving it to form trypsin. The free trypsin then cleaves the rest of the trypsinogen and chymotrypsinogen to their active forms.

Pancreatic secretions accumulate in intralobular ducts that drain the main pancreatic duct, which drains directly into the duodenum. Due to the importance of its enzyme contents, injuring the pancreas is a very dangerous situation. A puncture of the pancreas tends to require careful medical intervention.

Endocrine: – Scattered among the acini are the endocrine cells of the pancreas, in groups called the islets of Langerhans. They are: Insulin-producing beta cells (50–80% of the islet cells) Glucagon-releasing alpha cells (15–20%) Somatostatin-producing delta cells (3–10%) Pancreatic polypeptide-containing PP cells (remaining %). The islets are a compact collection of endocrine cells arranged in clusters and cords and are crisscrossed by a dense network of capillaries. The capillaries of the islets are lined by layers of endocrine cells in direct contact with vessels, and most endocrine cells are in direct contact with blood vessels, by either cytoplasmic processes or by direct apposition.

Liver: – The **liver** is an organ in vertebrates, including human. It plays a major role in metabolism and has a number of functions in the body including glycogen storage, plasma protein synthesis, and drug detoxification. It also produces bile, which is important in digestion. It performs and regulates a wide variety of high-volume biochemical reaction requiring specialized tissues.

Liver normally weighs between 1.3 – 3.0 kilograms and is a soft, pinkish-brown "boomerang shaped" organ. It is the second largest organ (the largest being the skin) and the largest gland within the human body. Its anatomical position in the body is immediately under the diaphragm on the right side of the upper abdomen. The liver lies on the right side of the stomach and makes a kind of bed for the gallbladder.

Liver is supplied by two main blood vessels on its right lobe: the hepatic artery and the portal vein. The hepatic artery normally comes off the celiac trunk. The portal vein brings venous blood from the spleen, pancreas, and small intestine, so that the liver can process the nutrients and byproducts of food digestion. The hepatic veins drain directly into the inferior vena cava.

The bile produced in the liver is collected in bile canaliculi, which merge from bile ducts. These eventually drain into the right and left hepatic ducts, which in turn merge to form the common hepatic duct. The cystic duct (from the gallbladder) joins with the common hepatic duct to form the common bile duct. Bile can either drain directly into the duodenum **via** the common bile duct or be temporarily stored in the gallbladder via the cystic duct. The common bile duct and the pancreatic duct enter the duodenum together at the ampulla of Vater. The branching's of the bile ducts resemble those of a tree, and indeed term "biliary tree" is commonly used in this setting.

The liver is among the few internal human organs capable of natural regeneration of lost tissue: as little as 25% of remaining liver can regenerate into a whole liver again. This is predominantly due to hepatocytes acting as unipotential stem cells. There is also some evidence of bio potential stem cells, called oval cell, which can differentiate into either hepatocytes or cholangiocytes (cells that line bile ducts).

Tracheo – esophageal fistula and esophageal atresia: Both of these conditions are congenital. In *Tracheo-esophageal fistula* there is a connection between the esophagus and the wind pipe (trachea) where there should not be one. In *Esophageal atresia* the esophagus of a newborn does not connect to the stomach but comes to a dead end right before the stomach. Both conditions require corrective surgery and are usually detected right after the baby is born. In some cases, it can be detected before the baby is born.

Esophagitis: – Esophagitis is inflammation of the esophagus and is a non-congenital condition. Esophagitis can be caused by certain medications or by infections. It can also be caused by gastro-esophageal reflux disease (GERD, a condition where the esophageal sphincter allows the acidic contents of the stomach to move back up into the esophagus. Gastro-esophageal reflux disease can be treated with medications, but it can also be corrected by changing what you eat.

Conditions Affecting Stomach and Intestines: Everybody has experienced constipation or diarrhea in their lifetime. With **constipation,** *the contents of the large intestines do not move along fast enough and waste material stays in the large intestines so long that almost all water is extracted out of the waste and it becomes hard.* With diarrhea you get the exact opposite reaction: *waste moves along too fast and the large intestines cannot absorb the water* before the waste is pushed through. Common flora bacteria assists in the prevention of many serious problems. Here are some more examples of common stomach and intestinal disorders:

Acute Appendicitis: – An exemplary case of acute appendicitis in a 10-year-old boy. The organ is enlarged and sausage-like (botuliform). This longitudinal section shows the angry red inflamed mucosa with its irregular luminal surface. Diagnosed and removed early in the course of the disease, this appendix does not show late complications, like transmural necrosis, perforation, and abscess formation. Appendicitis is the inflammation of the appendix, the finger-like pouch that extends from the cecum. The most common symptoms are abdominal pain, loss of appetite, fever, and vomiting. Children and teenagers are the most common victims of appendicitis, which must be corrected by surgery. While mild cases may resolve without treatment, most require removal of the inflamed appendix, either by laparotomy or laparoscopy. Untreated, mortality is high, mainly due to peritonitis and shock.

Celiac Disease: Celiac disease is a disorder in which a person's digestive system is damaged by the response of the immune system to a **protein called gluten,** which is found in **rye, wheat, and barley, and also in foods like breakfast cereal** and **pizza crust.** People who have celiac disease experience abdominal pain, diarrhea, bloating, exhaustion, and depression when they eat foods with gluten in them. They also have difficulty digesting their food. Celiac disease runs in families and becomes active after some sort of stress, like viral infections or surgery. The symptoms can be managed by following a gluten free diet. Doctors can diagnose this condition by taking a full medical history or with a blood test.

Diverticulitis: – Benign Gastric Ulcer: Diverticulitis is a common disease of the bowel, in particular the large intestine. Diverticulitis develops from diverticulosis, which involves the formation of pouches (diverticula) on the outside of the colon. Diverticulitis results if one of these diverticula becomes inflamed. In complicated diverticulitis, bacteria may subsequently infect the outside of the colon if an inflamed diverticula bursts open. If the infection spreads to the lining of the abdominal cavity (peritoneum), this can cause a potentially fatal peritonitis. Sometimes inflamed diverticula can cause narrowing of the bowel, leading to an obstruction. Also, the affected part of the colon could adhere to the bladder or other organ in the pelvic cavity, causing a fistula, or abnormal communication between the colon and an adjacent organ.

Gastritis and Peptic ulcers: Pain and bleeding. Medications are the best way to treat this condition. Usually the stomach and the duodenum are resistant to irritation because of the strong acids produced by the stomach. But sometimes a bacteria called Helicobacter pylori or the chronic use of drugs or certain medications, weakens the mucous layer that coats the stomach and the duodenum, allowing acid to get through the sensitive lining beneath. This can cause irritation and inflammation of the lining of the stomach, which is called gastritis, or cause peptic ulcers, which are holes or sores that form in the lining of the stomach and duodenum.

Gastrointestinal Infections: Gastrointestinal infections can be caused by bacteria such as Campylobacter, Salmonella, E. coli, or Shigella. They can also be caused by viruses or by intestinal parasites like amebiasis and Giardiasis. The most common symptoms of gastrointestinal infections are abdominal pain and cramps, diarrhea, and vomiting. These conditions usually go away on their own and don't need medical attention.

Inflammatory Bowel Disease: Inflammatory bowel disease is the chronic inflammation of the intestines, which usually affects older children, teens and adults. There are two major types, *ulcerative colitis* and *Crohn's disease* and indeterminate colitis, which occurs in 10–15% of patients. Ulcerative colitis usually affects just the rectum and large intestine, while Crohn›s disease can affect the whole gastrointestinal tract from mouth to anus along with some other parts of the body. Patients with these diseases also suffer from extra-intestinal symptoms including joint pain and red eye, which can signal a flare of the disease. These diseases are treated with medications and if necessary, Intravenous or IV feeding, or in the more serious cases, surgery to remove the damaged areas of the intestines.

Polyp: – A polyp is an abnormal growth of tissue (tumor) projecting from a mucous membrane. If it is attached to the surface by a narrow elongated stalk it is said to be pedunculated. If no stalk is present it is said to be sessile. Polyps are commonly found in the colon, stomach, nose, urinary bladder and uterus. They may also occur elsewhere in the body where mucous membranes exist like the cervix and small intestine.

DISORDERS OF THE PANCREAS, LIVER & GALLBLADDER

Disorders of the pancreas, liver, and gallbladder affect the ability to produce enzymes and acids that aid indigestion, examples of these disorders are.

Cystic Fibrosis: – Cystic fibrosis is a chronic, inherited illness where the production of abnormally thick mucous blocks the duct or passage ways in the pancreas and prevents the digestive fluids from entering the intestines, making it difficult for the person with the disorder to digest protein and fats, which cause important nutrients to pass through without being digested. People with this disorder take supplements and digestive enzymes to help manage their digestive problems.

Hepatitis: – Hepatitis is a viral condition that inflames a person's liver which can cause it to lose its ability to function. Viral hepatitis, like hepatitis A, B, and C, is extremely contagious. Hepatitis A, which is a mild form of hepatitis, can be treated at home, but more serious cases that involve liver damage, might require hospitalization.

Cholecystitis: – Acute or chronic inflammation if the gallbladder causes abdominal pain. 90% of cases of acute cholecystitis are caused by the presence of gallstones. The actual inflammation is due to secondary infection with bacteria of an obstructed gallbladder, with the obstruction caused by the gallstones. Gallbladder conditions are very rare in kids and teenagers but can occur when the kid or teenager has sickle cell anemia or in kids being treated with long term medications.

Cholecystitis – Biliary colic: This is when a gallstone blocks either the common bile duct or the duct leading into it from the gallbladder. This condition causes severe pain in the right upper abdomen and sometimes through to the upper back. It is described by many doctors as the most severe pain in existence, between childbirth and a heart attack. Other symptoms are nausea, vomiting, diarrhea, bleeding caused by continual vomiting, and dehydration caused by the nausea and diarrhea. Another more serious complication is total blockage of the bile duct which leads to jaundice, which if it is not corrected naturally or by surgical procedure can be fatal, as it causes liver damage. The only long term solution is the removal of the gallbladder.

Gastrointestinal dysfunctions: As we age, the amount of digestive enzymes produced by the body drops way down. This leads to decreased and slower digestion, slower absorption of nutrients and increased accumulation of feacal mater in the intestinal tract. Undigested food material and metabolic waste can also build up due to slow elimination, starting a series of health problems.

When digestion slows, it turns the intestines into a toxic environment. Helpful organisms cannot live in toxic environments. When the beneficial organisms die they are replaced by harmful organisms, such as yeasts and parasites, the most common being *Candida albicans*. This leads to changes in the intestinal wall which produce *leaky gut syndrome*, which allows many toxic chemicals to be introduced into the bloodstream. As a result, the entire toxic load of the body is increased, causing a bigger burden on the liver, kidneys and other body organs. When this happens the organs that are normally used for eliminating waste and supplying nutrients to the GI tract become a large dump for waste. This problem can be made worse by the use of prescriptions and over-the-counter medications, antibiotics, and a diet that is too low in fiber or contains 'junk food'.

Most people never think about their GI tract. We are concerned about what the outside of our bodies look like, but we completely ignore the inside. Because our bodies a very resilient, deterioration of the digestive system can go on for years with no symptoms or side-effects. When symptoms finally do appear they are usually very non-specific, and include: decreased energy, headaches, diarrhea, constipation, heartburn, and acid reflux. Over the years these symptoms become more serious, including: asthma, food allergies, arthritis, and cancer.

Poor digestion, poor absorption, and bacterial imbalance can be traced to many chronic conditions. Every organ in the body receives nutrients from the GI tract; if the GI tract is malfunctioning then the whole body suffers.

It is possible to return good health to GI tract by improving digestion, consuming the right amount of fiber, and cutting out junk food and refined sugars.

Improvement of the function of intestines is possible by taking fiber supplements and vitamins (especially B12 and vitamin K). Some doctors suggest herbal or vitamin enemas to cleanse and relieve constipation and to help stimulate *peristaltic movement* which will help to move the bowels.

Irritable Bowel Syndrome (IBS): Irritable Bowel Syndrome (IBS) is a disorder with symptoms that are most commonly bloating, abdominal pain, cramping, constipation, and diarrhea. IBS causes a lot of pain and discomfort. It does not cause permanent damage to the intestines and does not lead to serious diseases such as cancer. Most of the people affected with IBS can control their symptoms with stress management, diet, and prescription medication. For others IBS can be debilitating, they may be unable to go to work, travel, attend social events or leave home for even short periods of time. About 20 percent of the adult population has some symptoms of **IBS**, making it one of the most common intestinal disorders diagnosed by physicians. **It is more common in men than women and in about 50 percent of people affected it starts at about age 35.**

Researchers have not found out what exactly causes IBS. One idea is that people with IBS have a large intestine (colon) that is sensitive to certain foods and stress. The immune system may also be involved. It has also been reported that *serotonin* is linked with normal GI functioning. 95 percent of the body›s serotonin is located in the GI tract (the other 5 percent is in the brain). People with IBS have diminished receptor activity, causing abnormal levels of serotonin in the GI tract. Because of this, IBS patients experience problems with bowel movement, motility, and the sensation having more sensitive pain receptors in their GI tract. Many IBS patients suffer from depression and anxiety which can make symptoms worse.

There is no cure for IBS, but medications are an important part of relieving symptoms. **Fiber supplements or laxatives are helpful for constipation.** Anti diarrhoeals such as Imodium can help with diarrhea. An antispasmodic is commonly prescribed for colon muscle spasms.

Gastrointestinal Stromal Tumor (GIST): Gastrointestinal Stromal Tumors or GIST is an uncommon type of cancer in the GI tract (esophagus, stomach, small intestine, and colon). These types of cancers begin in the connective tissue like fat, muscles, nerves, cartilage, etc.

GIST: originates in the stroma cells. Stroma cells are strung along the GI tract and are part of the system that helps the body to know when to move food through the digestive system. Over half of GISTs occur in the stomach. Most cases occur in people between the ages of forty and eighty, but they can also occur in a person of any age.

All GISTs: of any size or location have the ability to spread. Even if a GIST is removed, it can reappear in the same area, or may even spread outside of the GI tract.

In the early stages, GIST is hard to diagnose because early-stage symptoms cannot be recognized. In the later stages a person can have vague abdominal pain, vomiting, abdominal bleeding that shows up in stool or vomit, low blood counts causing anemia, and having an early feeling of being full, causing a decrease in appetite.

GIST: Is now recognized as an aggressive cancer that is able to spread to other parts of the body. People who have been diagnosed with GIST should get treatment as soon as possible.

Food Allergies: Food allergies occur when the immune system thinks that a certain protein in any kind of food is a foreign substance and will try to fight against it.

Only about eight percent of children and two percent of adults actually have a food allergy. A person can be allergic to any kind of food, but the most common **food allergies are to nuts, cow's milk, eggs, soy, fish, and shellfish.** Most people who have a food allergy are allergic to fewer than four different foods.

The most common signs of food allergies are hives, swelling, itchy skin, itchiness, tingling or swelling in the mouth, coughing, trouble breathing, diarrhea, and vomiting. The two most common chronic illness that are associated with food allergies are eczema and asthma. Food allergies can be fatal if they cause the reaction called anaphylaxis. This reaction makes it hard for the person to breathe. This can be treated by an epinephrine injection.

Constipation: Not everyone is on the same schedule for having a bowel movement. Depending on the person, a "normal" schedule can range anywhere from three times a day to three times a week. If you start having bowel movements less than your own personal schedule, then you might be getting the signs of constipation.

When there is trouble in bowel movements it is considered as Constipation. The stool is very hard, making it difficult to pass leads to put strain. This may also feel like to have a bowel movement frequently.

During digestion of food, the waste products go through intestines by the muscle contractions. In the large intestine, most of the water and salt from the waste products are reabsorbed because they are needed by the body for everyday functions. One *can become constipated if too much water is absorbed, or if waste products move too slowly.*

Not getting enough fluids, a low fiber diet, age, not being physically active, depression, stress and pregnancy can all contribute to constipation. Medications and narcotics can also cause a person to get constipated. Chronic constipation may be a symptom of a liver problem such as a urea cycle disorder.

The best way for a person to treat constipation is to make sure that they are getting enough fluids as well as fiber in their diet. By doing this, the bulk of their stool is increased and made softer, so that it can move through the intestines more easily. Being more active and increasing daily exercise also helps keep bowel movements regulated.

Hemorrhoids: Are also known as haemorrhoids, emerods, or piles – are **varicosities** or **swelling and inflammation of veins** in the rectum and anus. Two of the most common types of hemorrhoids are external and internal hemorrhoids.

External Hemorrhoids: Are those that occur outside of the anal verge (the distal end of the anal canal). They are sometimes painful, and can be accompanied by swelling and irritation. Itching, although often thought to be a symptom from external hemorrhoids, is more commonly due to skin irritation. If the vein ruptures and a blood clot develops, the hemorrhoid becomes a **thrombosed hemorrhoid.**

Internal Hemorrhoids: Are those that occur inside the rectum. As this area lacks pain sensory receptor/receptors, *internal hemorrhoids are usually not painful and most people are not aware that they have them.* Internal hemorrhoids, however, may bleed when irritated. Untreated internal hemorrhoids can lead to two severe forms of hemorrhoids: prolapsed and strangulated hemorrhoids.

Prolapsed Hemorrhoids: Are internal hemorrhoids that are so distended that they are pushed outside of the anus. If the anal sphincter muscle goes into spasm and traps a prolapsed hemorrhoid outside of the anal opening, the supply of blood is cut off, and the hemorrhoid becomes a **strangulated hemorrhoid.**

Bleeding in the Gastrointestinal tract: Bleeding in the gastrointestinal tract doesn't always mean you have a disease, it's usually a symptom of a digestive problem. The cause of the bleeding may not be that serious, it could be something that can be cured or controlled such as hemorrhoids. However, locating the source of the bleeding is very important. The gastrointestinal tract contains many important organs like the esophagus, stomach, small intestine, large intestine or colon, rectum, and anus. *Bleeding can come from one or more of these area from a small ulcer in the stomach, or a large surface like the inflammation of the colon.* Sometimes a person doesn't even know they are bleeding. When this happens, it is called hidden, or occult bleeding. Simple tests can detect hidden blood in the stool When this happens, it is called hidden, or occult bleeding. Simple tests can detect hidden blood in the stool.

What Causes Bleeding in the Digestive Tract: Esophageal bleeding may be caused by Mallory-Weiss syndrome which is a tear in the esophagus. Mallory-Weiss syndrome is usually caused by excessive vomiting or may be caused by childbirth, a hiatal hernia, or increased pressure in the abdomen caused by coughing. Various medications can cause stomach ulcers or inflammations. *Medications containing aspirin or alcohol, and various other medications(mainly those used for arthritis) are some examples of these.* **Benign tumors or cancer** of the stomach may also cause bleeding. These disorders don't usually produce massive bleeding. *The most common source of bleeding usually occurs from ulcers in the duodenum.* **Researchers believe that these ulcers are caused by excessive stomach acid and a bacteria called Helicobacter Pylori.** In the lower digestive tract, the most common source of bleeding is in the large intestine, and the rectum. Hemorrhoids are the most common cause of bleeding in the digestive tract. Hemorrhoids are enlarged veins in the anal area which produces bright red blood that you see in the toilet or on the toilet paper.

How to Recognize Bleeding in the Digestive Tract: The signs of bleeding in the digestive tract vary depending on the site and severity of the bleeding. If the **blood** is coming **from the rectum**, it would be bright **red blood**. If it was coming from higher up in the **colon or from**

the small intestine, the blood would be **darker**. When the blood is coming **from the stomach, esophagus, or the duodenum**, the stool would be **black and tarry**.

If the bleeding is hidden, or occult, a person may not notice changes in the stool color. If extensive bleeding occurs, a person may feel dizzy, faint, weak, short of breath, have diarrhea or cramp abdominal pain. Shock can also occur along with rapid pulse, drop in blood pressure, and difficulty urinating. Fatigue, lethargy, and pallor from anemia will settle in if the bleeding is slow. Anemia is when the blood's iron-rich substance, hemoglobin, is diminished.

HOW THE BLEEDING IN THE DIGESTIVE TRACT IS DIAGNOSED?

To diagnose bleeding in the digestive tract the bleeding must be located and a complete history and physical are very important. Here are some of the procedures that diagnose the cause of bleeding.

An endoscopy is a common diagnostic technique that allows direct viewing of the bleeding site. Since the endoscope can detect lesions and confirm the complaint

Common Causes of Bleeding in the Digestive Tract: Hemorrhoids – Gastritis (inflammation) – Inflammation (ulcerative colitis) – Colo rectal Polyps – Colo rectal Cancer – Duodenal Ulcer – Enlarged Veins – Esophagiti (inflammation of the esophagus) – Mallory – Weiss Syndrome – Ulcers Iron and beets can also turn the blood red or black giving a false indication of blood in the stool.

HOW TO RECOGNIZE BLOOD IN THE STOOL AND VOMIT ?

(a) Bright red blood coating the stool (b) Dark blood mixed with the stool (c) Black or tarry stool (d) Bright red blood in the vomit (e) Grainy appearance in vomit

SYMPTOMS OF ACUTE BLEEDING

Weakness – – Shortness of breath – Dizziness – – Cramp abdominal pain – – Feeling light headed – – Diarrhea

SYMPTOMS OF CHRONIC BLEEDING

Fatigue – – Shortness of breath—Lethargy – – Pallor

Case Study: Bob had a history of chronic pain in his intestinal area, and wasn't sure what it was. His doctor suspected what it was and gave Bob antibiotics, which helped. It so happened that whenever Bob ate popcorn or nuts he would get this pain. Sometimes it would just go away, other times he had to go on antibiotics. The doctor ordered some tests, and told Bob he would have to stay away from nuts, popcorn, tomatoes, strawberries, and anything else with seeds or hard parts; something in his bowels couldn't tolerate those foods. Bob ate a pretty healthy diet so he couldn't understand what was happening. A few years later, Bob had another series of painful episodes. The pain was so great Bob could hardly stand, let alone go to work. This time the doctor did more tests and found out that his lower intestine was almost blocked. Surgery was ordered. What did Bob have?

GLOSSARY

Amebiasis: An inflammation if the intestines caused by infestation with Entameba histolytica (a type of ameba) and characterized by frequent loose stools flecked with blood and mucus.

B12: A vitamin important for the normal formation of red blood cells and the health of the nerve tissues. Undetected and untreated B12 deficiency can lead to anemia and permanent nerve and brain damage

Chemical digestion: Is a chemical breakdown of food when being in the mouth (oral cavity). Is the digestive secretions of saliva that moistens food and introduces gastric juices and enzymes that are produced in the stimulation to certain macronutrients, such as, carbohydrates. In this, the mouth saliva carries an enzyme called amylase for breaking down carbohydrates.

Crohn's Disease: Described as skip lesions in the large and small bowel it is a **malabsorption disorder** that can affect the gastrointestinal tract from the mouth to the anus.

Deamination: When an amino acid group breaks off an amino acid that makes a molecule of ammonia and keto acid.

Lipase: An enzyme produced by microorganisms that split the fat molecules into fatty acids which create flavour

Mechanical digestion: The crushing of the teeth and rhythms made by the movement of the tongue, the teeth aid in tearing and pulverizing food, while the tongue helps with peristalsis (movement), of food down the esophagus.

Chapter–4 on "Anatomy & Physiology of Digestive Tract" highlights its operation, mal functions, and peculiar symptoms. **Hence the Physician should study in depth so as to aim at the selection of correct remedy.**

CHAPTER – 6

PROCESS OF DIGESTION

Study the "Surface Anotomy of Abdomen, details of each region of Digestive Tract to acquaint with the structures of abdomen to achieve perfect treatment of the complaint.

THE SURFACE ANATOMY OF ADOMEN

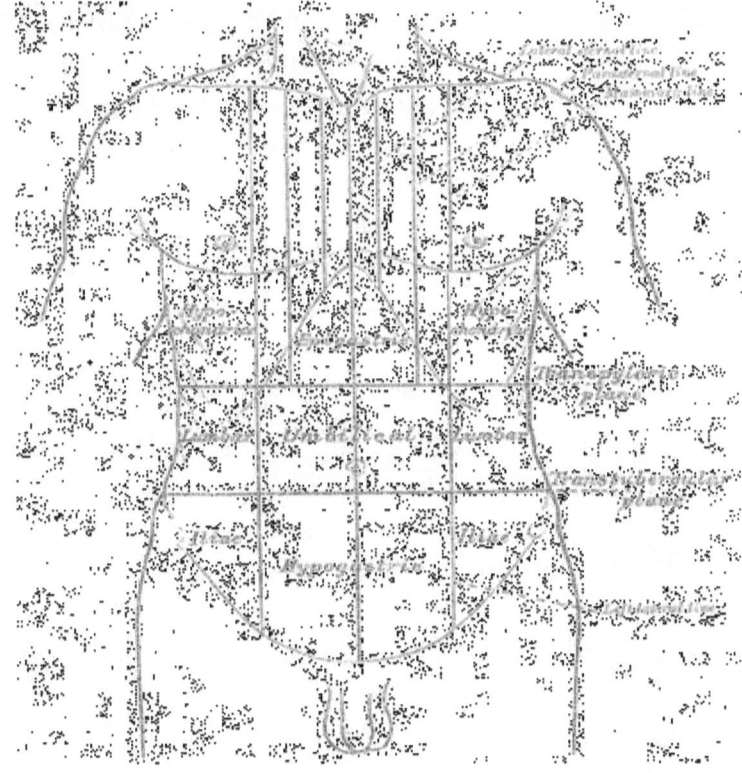

BRIEF DETAILS OF EACH REGION

LEFT	CENTRE	RIGHT
Left Hypochondrium Consist of part of fundus and body of the stomach the spleen and tail of the pancreas, the splenic flexure of the colon, upper half of the left kidney and left supra renal	Epigastric region The left lobe and lobules spigelic of the liver	Right Hypchondrium The right lobe of the liver and the gall bladder, and the right suprarenal
Left Lumbar Descending colon, part of the omentum, lower part of the left kidney and some convolutions of the small intestines.	Umbilical region The middle and pyloric end of the stomach. The first, second & paroximal position of the third part of the pancreas, the middle of the transverse colon, part of the great omentum ad mesentery & some convolutions of the jejunam and ileum	Right lumbar The and proximal part of the transverse colon, lower part of the right kidney, and some convolutions of the small intestine
Left Iliac Sigmoid flexure of the colon, ureter and ovary	Hypogastrium Convolutions of the small intestines and bladder in children and in adults liver distended, the appendix, the pelvic colon, and the uterus during pregnancy	Right iliac The calcium, ovary and ureter

DIGESTIVE TRACT

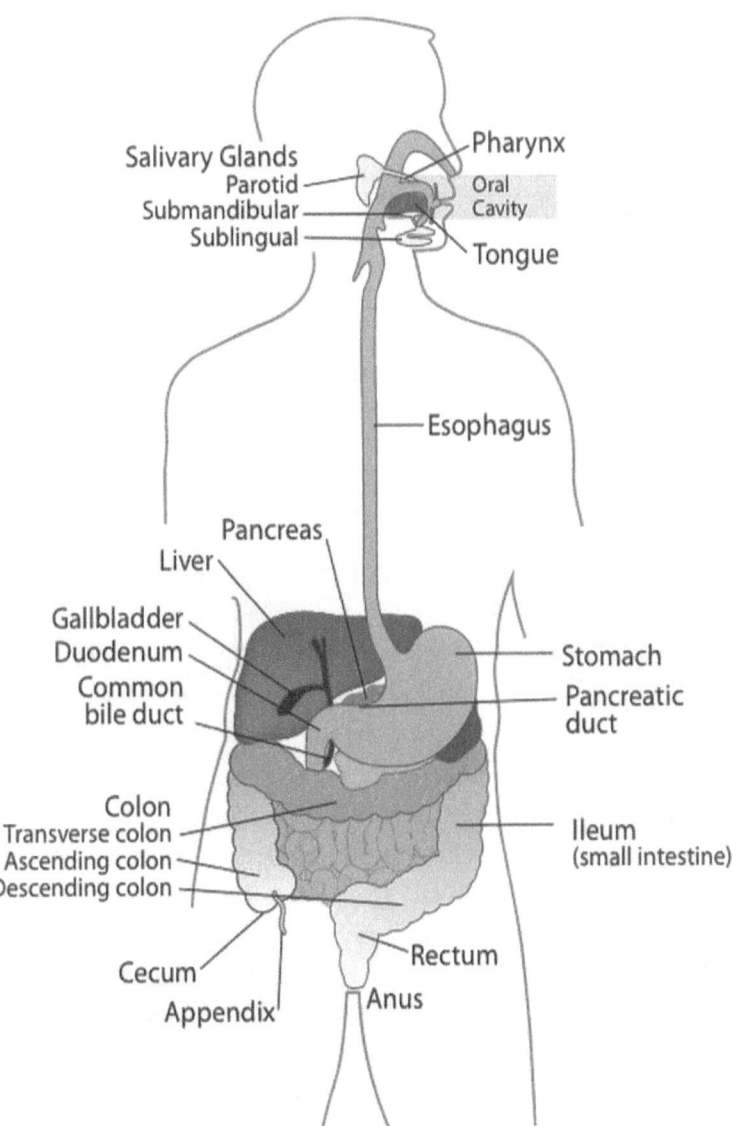

Digestion is considered effective when the food taken is assimilated effectively and converted into blood without the conscious of patient about any part of the digestive tract.

Go through below the points in relation to the Alimentary Canal outline of the Digestive Tract depicted above

Pain relation	To be checked
Pain at the lower portion of oesophagus i.e. it can be at epigastria (Gastro Esophagul – Refer disease GERD)	May be trouble with cardiac orifice of Stomach GERD (Gastro Esophagul Disease)
Pain in the stomach immediately after eating or during eating	(a) Gastric origin – (b) Acidity – Hyperacidity (c) Erosions or Ulcer – Duration of pain can be for two or half hours i.e. till the food leaves the stomach
Pain after 2/4 hours of eating (Location Right side)	It may be due to erosion of Duodenum/Pyloric junction or Ulcer – The duration of pain (I) after two & half hours may continue to 4 hours – total time – It can also be suspected at jejunal region – (2" to 3") (ll) Intestine when extended to left side line of abdomen – can be due to erosion or Ulcer of Jejunum.
Pain after 4 to 5 hours after eating	Related to small intestine where there can be strictures/ulcers/inflammation (enteritis) or cam be due to flatulency – The pain may continue for say 3 to 4 hours i.e. till the food leaves small intestine and absorption takes place.
Pain after 7 to 8 hours after eating	(a) By that time the food reaches large intestines through caceum (Ascending colon) – if so, pain is felt on right side i.e. can be appendicitis. (b) If the pain is in the transverse region of Abdomen i.e. below the diaphragm. may be due to Ulceration or inflammation, erosion or catarrh of transverse column. c) If the pain is felt on the left side of abdomen it can be due to inflammation/ erosion of descending column

	Journey of Food through Digestive Tract
1.	Description/function/and feeling and the part(s) of the Digestive tract involved – Secretions developed – with the time taken towards each
2.	Transit time to pass through the gut from mouth to anus in a healthy adult transit time is about 24–72 hours
3.	Before eating: Sights, sounds and smells of food Digestive activity begins with the sights, and smells of food. Just looking at or smelling appetising food can result in the brain sending signals to the *salivary glands* to make the mouth water and to the *stomach* to secrete gastric juice. The human has an important role in the perception of colour, and this influences out idea of food flavour.
4.	**Chewing: Ingestion – 1** Chewing mechanically mixes food with saliva from the Salivary glands, Amylase in saliva chemically digests starch in the food. The mixing process is lubricated by mucin, a slippery protein in saliva. Each mouthful takes approximately 3–60 seconds.
5.	**Swallowing: Ingestion – 2** The food is formed into a small ball called a *bolus,* which is pushed to the back of the mouth by the tongue. Involuntary *muscle* contraction in the pharynx, the **bolus goes** down towards the oesophagus. This *swallowing reflex* takes about 1–3 seconds
6.	**Periastalsis: Ingestion – 3** In the oesophagus, the bolus is moved along in rhythmic contractions of the muscles present in the walls. For a medium-sized bolus, it takes about 5–8 seconds to reach the stomach.
7.	**Time to empty: Stomach** Food is mixed with gastric juice. Strong muscular contractions in the stomach wall reduce the food to **chime** – thick material. The pyloric sphincter at the lower end of the stomach slowly releases **chime** into the duodenum. Emptying the stomach takes 2 – 6 hours.

Continued...

8.	**Absorption: Jejunum**
	Peristaltic waves of muscular *contraction* mix and move the chime down the duodenum and into the *jejunum*. It has a huge surface area created by finger-like structures called villi. These assist with the absorption of the end products of digestion into the bloodstream.
9.	**Absorption: Illeum**
	By the time chime has reached the ileum, most of the digestion processes involving *carbohydrate* protein and fats have occurred. Its main function is to absorb the end products of digestion and release *hormones* that regulate feelings of fullness.
10.	**Elapsed time: Ileocaecal valve**
	Undigested remains of food are passed through a one-way muscular valve into the first part of the *large intestine* known the *caecum* – a small pouch that acts as a temporary storage site. By the time food remains have reached this point, about 5–12 hours have elapsed.
11.	**Colon time: Large intestine**
	The large intestine is 1.5 – 1.8m in length and is divided into the caecum, *colon* and *rectum*. The colon is further divided into 4 parts – ascending colon, descending colon and sigmoid colon. The large intestine consists of the caecum, colon, rectum and anal canal. It is about 1.5 metres long and has an average diameter of about 6 cm. The 4 major functions of the large intestine are recovery of water and electrolytes, formation and storage of faeces and fermentation some of the indigestible food matter by bacteria.
12.	**Fermentation at Colon:**
	Slower peristaltic movements push undigested food remains along the colon, which mix freely with the resident bacterial population. The bacteria ferment of the food remains, producing *short-chain fatty acids* as well other important *chemicals* such

13.	Mass shift: Sigmoid colon
	The liquid from the small intestine changes into a semi-solid form known as a stool. The sigmoid colon temporarily stores the stool until a mass movement empties it into the rectum. Residence time in the colon ranges from 4–72 hours, with a normal average of 36 hours.
14.	Egestion: Rectum
	The rectum's external opening, the anus, is controlled by a set of muscles. When filled with a mass movement from the sigmoid colon, the rectum is stretched and produces the desire to defecate. If inhibited to live in, the urge to defecate subsides but returns several hours later (Constipation?).

Recollection of various states towards the journey of food from mouth to anus, to infer the results towards Defective functions at each step and how it leads to complaints, accordingly. **This can ease the Physician for selection of correct remedy.**

Chewing ingestion starts at mouth with the help of teeth and tongue whereat saliva, with water, mucus, amylase, lipase and sodium bicardonate is produced from the salivary glands i.e. structures found in and around the mouth and throat that produce saliva. The major salivary glands are the parotid, sub-mandibular and sublingual. **Amylase** – an enzyme present in saliva that can digest starch. – **Starch** – A complex carbohydrate found chiefly in seeds, fruits, tubers, root s and stem pith of plants. Commonly found in foods, such as potatoes, wheat, rice and corn.

Bolus: The final stage food after chewing is formation of bolus which is ready to swallow:

INFERENCE HERE

Digestion activity first begins at **BRAIN** which send signals to all the parts in the mouth towards taste, preference of food selection etc.

and then only it is successfully ends till the stage of **bolus** and make it ready for swallowing. If the very first Chewing ingestion adopted " *in a hurried mood, with lack of interest, or otherwise when mind is in tension, the **bolus** formed in the mouth may be **defective**, which may affect on further **ingestions also** upto the Rectum. Such defective Bolus may produce adverse results/ailments i.e. in the entire Digestive tract.*

Here one should note that all the secretions in the mouth are ALKALINE which help in neutralisation of excessive Hydrochloric acid produced in the Gastric region and reduce creation of Gastro Acidic disorders leading to i.e. burning sensation, erosions in the Gastric internal layers thereby allowing the H – Pylori infection to enter below such eroded layers ending in Peptic Ulcers starting from Eseophagus, Cardiac end of the Stomach, Pyloric region to Intestines, etc. Similarly, **whereas in the defective Chew Ingestion and Bolus formation may not contain ALKALINE property the reasons for which are narrated above.**

This is why our elders suggest repeatedly that one should keep their mind peaceful while taking food, so as to ensure perfect digestion of food consumed, whereas it is kept for deaf ear right from youth to middle aged.

IF SO WHAT ABOUT OTHER COMPLAINTS?

All of us agree that a perfect digestive system of the Human Body, converts the food into basic blood and supply to Circulatory System, and moved to the same to Respiratory System for its purification. The perfect Digestive System has inbuilt immunity system so as to combat with various infections in it. Towards Acute infections remedies are available in all types of medical systems though the concept of treatment may differ in each type.

The **HEART** located in the centre of Circulatory System is very sophisticated motor for successful Circulation even to the minute nook & corner of all parts of the Human Body. It receives impure blood through **veins** and send to the Resparative Tract for its purification and receive the purified blood from the Resperative Tract through **arteries,** so as to supply through out the body. **This cycle of circulation continues day and night and life long.**

An evil thinking in the Mind tries to adopt evil operation which obviously produce evil result. **HOMOEOPATHY believes on the above concept as Mind is responsible in the beginning, to end in evil/ negative results.** In other words when the Mind is disturbed, most of the functions of various parts of human body are also affected, ultimately leading to many complaints, even **immunity mechanism in the body is not an exception** – as it may create an incapability to combat with various infections from time to time.

If the readers wish to know to get considerable details on Homoeopathy other than at **CHAPTER – I** and **II** of this book, they may indent for the printed copy of "**Handbook For Homoeopathy**" written by the Author through **amazon.in, flipkart.com, or infibeam.com**

In a condensed way, we will go through the parts of Digestive Tract and on secretions related to them. (Refer the figure of Digestive Tract)

Oesophagus: A thin muscular–walled tube that runs from mouth to stomach. Also known as the gullet, it allows food to be transport to the stomach by peristaltic muscular movement.

Swallowing Reflex: Swallowing, also known as deglultition, is the process that makes something pass from the mouth, to the pharynx, into oesophagus and then to the stomach. It is a complex neuromuscular process involving voluntary actions (mouth) followed by involuntary actions (pharynx) and peristalsis (oesophagus).

Chyme: A creamy paste formed after food in the stomach has been mixed and churned with gastric juice over a period of time.

Pyloric Sphincter: A muscular valve that controls the release of food from the stomach into the duodenum.

Duodenum: The first section of the human small intestine, It is about 25–30 cm in length and plays vital role in the digestion of food into it from the stomach.

Small intestine: That part of the gastrointestinal tract that connects the stomach to the large intestine. It consists of three parts, the duodenum, the jejunam and the ileum. Ileum is the last of Small intestine (about 3 m long in human). It links to the large intestine.

Villi: (Singular: Villus) Thin fingure – like structure that project from the internal lining of the jejunum and ileum. They greatly increase the surface area of the small intestine, allowing for rapid absorption of the products of digestion into blood stream.

Surface area: The total area of the surface of a three – dimentional object.

Enzyme: A complex protein that acts as a catalyist (speeds up chemical reactions) in specific biochemical reactions. For example, saliva contains an enzyme amylase that can breakdown starch into simple sugars.

Digestion: The mechanical and chemical breaking down food into smaller components that can be absorbed into a blood stream.

Pancreas: A greyish-pink organ, about 15 cm long, that stretches across the back of the abdomen, behind the stomach. It produces hormones such as insulin and glucogen (endocrine function) as well as pancreatic juice that contains digestive enzyme (exocrine function)

Gall Bladder: A small pouch-like that sits just beneath the liver. It stores bile produced by the liver and releases it into the duodenum during the digestion of food.

Contraction: 1. The shortening of an object 2. when muscles become shorter and pull.

Jejunum: The middle section of the small intestine, about 2–3 m in lenth, where chemical breakdown of food is completed.

Carbohydrate: Any of a large group of energy – producing compounds, including sugars and starches and starches, that contain carbon, hydrogen and oxygen.

Hormone: A chemical substance secreted by an endocrine gland into the bloodstream. It acts on specific target cells to produce a given response control and regulate the activity of certain cells or organs.

Large Intestine: The end part of the gastrointestinal tract that includes the caecum, colon and rectum.

Caecum: A pouch connecting the last part of the small intestine, called the ileum. The first part of the colon, known as the ascending colon.

Colon: That part of the Large Intestine between the caecum and rectum. It consists of four sections: the ascending colon, the transverse colon, the descending colon and the sigmoid colon.

Rectum: The end of the Large intestine, about 12 cm in humans, that temporarily stores faeces prior to ejection.

Visceral drainage remedies:

When a selected similimum fails to respond and where the following parts are involved in alimentary tract troubles, try one of the following drainage remedies in Mother tincture (Q) as stated by Charles C Boericke.

Liver – Cardus Mar

Mucus Membranes – Inula

Spleen: Helianthias: –

CHAPTER – 7

AILMENTS OF DIGESTIVE TRACT – TREATMENT

After we have gone through **Process of Digestion**, let us proceed towards treatment of ailments, its symptoms, with *Homoeopathy Remedies.*

Digestive Tract is a major part of human body which convert the food to such a minute form so as to convert it into blood and extend energy to all the parts of human body.

The list of remedies together with symptoms are given in **Anatomical order of Digestive Tract**: i.e. from **Mouth to Rectum**. In all cases the remedies are used in 30th potency – otherwise in the specific potency wherever mentioned.

Before taking up treatment with remedies, it should be found whether the complaint can be treated with auxiliary methods, like timely food habits, regulation of diet, avoiding food articles/drinks aggravating the ailments etc. as far as possible.

Note: Almost in all the cases, the remedies are to be used in 30 potency except otherwise stated: < Indicate aggravation – > amelioration

MOUTH

Stomatitis – Inflammation in the mouth – Remedies	
Arum Triph.	Very sore feeling in the mouth, redness of tongue elevated papillae, lips and corners of mouth cracked, sore nose.
Ars.Alb.	Is indicated in livid and bluish aphthea with blisters in the mouth and on tongue – Gangrenous stomatitis of the cheek and gums with fever – Black spurt in ulcerative portion – Intense restlessness and prostration.
Aethusa	Has general aphthous conditions of the mouth and throat with difficulty in swallowing – child ejects the milk in large curds owing to bad stomach – vomiting is spurting in character and attended by prostration.
Alumen	Ulceration an dryness of the mouth – Thirst for cold water
Borax	The mucus membrane looks shrivelled as if burnt – Dryness of mouth – Stomatitis with thirst and vomiting – The blisters bleed easily on touch
Belladonna	Dry, red, burning – Thirstless
Capscicum	Simple inflammation of the mouth with burning
Hepar Sulph	Scurfy patches at mouth corners, pimples on chin – Ulcers of the palate which eat away the uvula, destroy the soft palate and later destroy osseous portion of the roof of the mouth – Extremely offensive smell from the mouth like that of spoiled cheese
Hydrocotyle	Flabby tongue, showing the imprint of teeth, with a feelings if it had been burnt, especially on the front part of the tongue.
Hydrastis	Specially beneficial in aphthous sore mouth – tongue heavily coated – follicular ulcers in the mouth – secretion of tenacious mucus from the month
Merc.sol.	Very useful in ulceration stomatitis where there is no history of abuse of mercury – Ulcerative gums with great saliva, offensive breath and night aggravation
Merc.cor.	Ulcerative inflammation of the month

Mur.Acid	Aphthous mouth, psoriasis of tongue, recurring ulcers
Nitric Acid	Saliva is acrid and offensive – excoriating the corners of the month – Teeth look yellow and are loose and drop out – it cures ulceration and gangrenous and chronic varieties – Foul smell from mouth
Nat. Mur.	Simple inflammation with mapped tongue and red insular patches – Mouth and tongue feel dry, hot and burnt
Psorinum	Tip of tongue dry and feels as if burnt
Phosphorus	Ulcerative stomatitis with bleeding from gums – white or yellow lines about the gums – general emaciation
Rheum	Mouth covered with offensive mucus after sleeping
Sepia	Pain in tongue as if burnt

Stomatitis –Bio-chemic remedies	
Calc. fluor	Gumboil, hard swellings on the jaws or gums. Indurations. Cold sores at corners of mouth.
Calc. Phos	Gums painful and inflamed in teething children. Pale appearance of the gums, sign of anaemia. Upper lip swollen and painful.
Calc. Sulph	Inside of lips sore, raw sores on lips. Gums bleed on brushing teeth.
Ferr. Phos	Gums sore, red, hot and inflamed. Tenderness, dryness or heat of the mucous membrane of the mouth.
Kali mur.	Aphthae, thrush, white ulcers in the mouths of little children or nursing mothers. Canker, ulcers of the mouth. Gum-boils, soft swelling before matters form, excoriation of the mouth. Great foetor from the mouth. The mouth is red and swollen, thick, watery secretions. Gums puffed, white or yellow in color. Gums bleed easily. Mucous patches. Syphilitic ulceration of gums. True gangrene of the the cheek.

Continued...

Nat. Mur.	Thrush with flow of saliva, salivation. Blisters like pearls around mouth. Lips swollen: eruptions on chin. Gumboil with throbbing and boring pains.
Nat. Phos.	This remedy has has few equals for ulceration of the buccal mucous membrane. "Canker sores" of the lips and cheeks yield t o this remedy in the 3X or 6X attenuation, where Borax, Ant im card, Baptiasia, Kali chlor, etc., hace failed to cure (S.J. of H)

PHARYNGITIS

ACUTE PHARYNGITIS SYNONYMS: SORE THROAT

An acute inflammation of the mucous membrane of pharynx. It may be associated with the acute inflammation of the tonsils, nares and of the palate.

Symptoms:

The mucous membrane is in dark red colour, swollen and is covered with a layer of mucus containing pus cells. If the congestion is extremely acute the mucus may contain blood. There is frequent desire to swallow, deglutition is painful, thereby there is tickling in the throat which may cause a dry cough, and the hacking which may give rise to vomiting. In some cases the constitutional symptoms are pronounced. There is a slight fever which does not last long. The duration of the attack is from two to six days.

ACUTE PHARYNGITIS – Remedies	
Aconite	Should be studied when there has been an exposure to cold. There is fever with arterial excitement and the throat is dry, and there is a sensation of pricking and burning referred to it
Apis Mel	There is oedema of the mucous surfaces, with painful and difficult swallowing attended with stinging pains.

Belladonna	Redness of the pharynx, soft palate, uvula and tonsils. The patient complains a sensation of dryness, constriction and difficult breathing. The face is flushed and hot
Capscicum	Throat [presents a dark red hue. The breath is fetid, uvula is elongated, there is sensation in the pharynx, and a dry burning sensation between the acts of deglution.
Gelsemium	Faeces are dry, irritated and burning. The tonsils are inflamed and there is a sensation of burning in the oesophagus. The patient is drowsy, face is flushed, pulse is small and the arterial tension is low.
Merc.iod. flavus	Throat is sore and painful swallowing. There is a constant secretion of saliva, difficult to dislodge, as a result causes retching. The mucus descends from the back of the nose to throat. Tongue is broad, flabby and with yellow coating, especially upon the back.
Nux Vom	There is a sensation in the throat as if were rough, raw, sore or scraped. There is a constant dry hacking cough that is attended with headache and pain in the hypochondria which is worse while coughing. There is soreness in the stomach and hypochondria. The patient is cross, irritable and is worse during the morning
Phytolacca	There is enlargement and soreness of the glands about the angle of the jaw. The mucous membranes are dark red swollen. There is difficulty in swallowing. There is aching and pain in the limbs.
Rhus Tox	There is a sensation of great debility, and a roughness of the pharynx. The fauces are oedematous, the uvula is elongated, puffed, translucent and has the appearance of jelly

CHRONIC PHARYNGITIS

There is a dull pain in the throat upon speaking or swallowing, and there may be hoarseness, a dry cough and tickling in the throat. The lymphoid of the pharynx are enlarged, raised above the surrounding surface and may coalesce. The small venules are dilated, and may rupture and thus cause streaks of blood in the expectorate material. A moderate degree of pharyngitis may give rise to no symptoms apart from the recurrent attacks. In other cases there is great distress in speaking, singing and a to degree when swallowing, which is always aggravated by a nervous condition that ensues. In some cases there is a neurosis established which is out of proportion to the organic disease, and mucus may accumulate in the naso-pharynx and lead to distress, hacking and vomiting. This may extend downward, resulting in hoarseness and aphonia.

CHRONIC PHARYNGITIS – Remedies	
Alumina	Mucous membranes are dry, glazed and red. The voice is hoarse, husky and weak, especially during the morning. There is a sensation of rawness and soreness of the throat and as if a splinter was sticking in the pharynx. There may be a small amount of mucus, but it is tenacious.
Aesculus Hip	There is great dryness, burning and scraping in the throat and posterior nares, with a sensation of excoriation and pricking, hawking and dropping of clear mucus into the throat with a tendency to constipation and haemorrhoids
Arg. Met	Chronic pharyngitis – Constant hoarseness, and as soon as the patient begins to talk or sing there is an easy expectoration of mucus that looks like starch paste.
Arg. Nit.	Chronic follicular pharyngitis when the parts present a dark red appearance, the patient hawks thick tenacious mucus from the throat and burning in the throat with a sensation of a splinter being lodged there.
Cal. Phos.	Young subjects who have grown rapidly and have glandular and tonsillar enlargement. The pharynx is studied with enlarged follicles and the whole pharyngeal tissue presents a condition hyperplasia. **Also compare Calc. Carb., Calc.Iod., Baryta Carb., Baryta Iod., Sulphur.**

Hydrastis	Hypertrophic catarrh, where there is swelling, redness and soreness of the pharynx. The mucus of a yellow colour and stringy.
Iodium	To scrofulous subjects who complain of a gradually increasing emaciation in spite of a good appetite.
Kali Iod.	Hoarsenesss, burning, scraping and roughness of the pharynx, pain in the chest, cough and oppression in breathing. The expectoration is greenish, stringy and salty.
Kali Mur.	There are adenoid vegetations and enlarged follicles. The mucous membrane between the follicles is pale, white and transparent discharge. There is Eustachian catarrh and deafness results. If the remedy is continued over a prolonged period it will be found to lessen susceptibility to acute attacks.
CHRONIC PHARYNGITIS – Remedies	
Nux Vom	For men who are addicted to the use of alcohol and tobacco. They are subject to gastric derangements and constipation with ineffectual urging to stool. The pharynx presents an alternation of atrophic white patches and enlarged follicles. The pharynx is exceedingly sensitive and there is gagging and retching whenever the tongue depressor is passed beyond the lips.
Sang. Nit.	Follicular pharyngitis where there is a sensation of burning, soreness, and rawness in the pharynx. The discharge is thick yellow and may contain traces of the blood.
Sang. Canad	The pharynx presents a red, congested appearance, and ulceration may be present. The patient complains of a sensation of burning and dryness of the pharynx which is not relieved by drinking water. There is a frontal headache, heat in the head, great dryness of the throat and paroxysms of coughing which are painful without expectoration.
Wyethia	Dryness of the throat with constant desire to swallow. Pharynx presents a dark red appearance and patient complains that it is sensitive, feels swollen dry and sensation of burning with a constant desire to clear the throat.

Continued...

Pharyngitis – Bio-chemic remedies	
Calc. Fluor	Relaxed condition of the uvala, tickling on the larynx. Exciting cough. Hawking of mucs early in morning. Burning in throat better by warmth. Follicular sore throat with plugs of mucus constantly forming on the tonsils.
Calc. phos	Clergyman's sore throat, as intercurrent.
Calc. Sulph	Supporting sore throat (see Tonsillitis), ulcerated sore throat, yellow matter, last stage.
Ferr.Phos	Throat dry, red, inflamed, with very much pain (very frequent doses), redness congestion, heat, fever, pain and throbbing in ulcerated sore throat, sore and inflamed palate, acute stage of laryngitis. Burning of the throat with pain. Sore throat of singers and those who use the voice daily.
Kali-Mur	When swelling of the glands or tonsils sets in, this remedy alternately with Ferr.Phos alterntely. Throat ulcerated with whitish or grayish patches or spots, and the chracterisitic white tongue. Syphilisitic sore throat; pain on swallowing. Hawks up offensive, cheesy small lumps. This remedy works as a wash and gargle in sore mouth and throat. **Glandular Pharyngitis**. Adenoid elevations; secretion mucus which is white and tough; also in posterior nares. Patient hawks and snuffs to get it out. In follicular Pharyngitis, with tough, tenacious secretion and cough, temporarily relieved by removal, after great effort, of the clinging sputa. There is dry ness, difficult and painful swallowing. Found it more frequently useful than *Kali bichromium.*
Kali phos	Gangrenous sore throat. Throat very dry; desire to swallow all the time. Salty mucus raised from throat.
Nat. Mur.	Enlargement of the throat. Goitre, if with watery secretions. Inflammation of the mucous lining of the throat, transparent mucus covering the parts, relaxed uvula. Chronic sore throat with feelling of plug or lump, and great dryness of throat. Constriction and stitches in the throat. Follicular pharyngitis, especially in smokers after nitrate of silver treatment.

Nat Phos	Tonsils coated with a yellow creamy mucus, raw feeling, moist deposit on the tongue mornings, looking yellow. Secretion as of a lump in the throat, worse swallowing liquid.

AILMENTS OF ESOPHAGUS

Conditions Affecting the Esophagus: There are two different types of conditions that may affect the esophagus. The **first** type is called **congenital:** meaning a person is born with it. The second type is called **non-congenital:** meaning the person develops it after birth. Some examples of these are: This is a muscular tube about 10 inches in length. It begins as a continuation of the pharynx, posterior to the cricoid cartilage and anterior to the sixth cervical vertebra. It enters the upper opening of the chest slightly to the left of the median line, descends to the esophageal opening in the diaphgram, and opens into the cardia of the stomach at the level of the tenth oeleventh dorsal vertebra.

Peptic ulcers of the Esophagus: These are rare. When they do occur they are situated near the cardia. They have sharp margins and are usually round. They are seldom recognized during life. The dangers are haemorrhages, perforation, cicatrisation with stenosis of the oesophagus and carcinomatous degeneration. The management is similar to that of gastric ulcer.

AILMENTS OF OESOPHAGUS – Remedies	
Aconite	Violent pain in middle of chest through into the back, < from; when swallowing it feels as if the food remained lodged in region of heart; lying on back impossible
Alumina	Sensation of constriction in oesophagus every time he swallows a mouthful of food; violent pressive pain, as if a portion of esophagus: were contracted or compressed in middle of chest, especially during deglution, but also WHEN NOT SWALLOWED, with oppression of chest, altenating with palpitation of heart, especially after a mea.

Continued...

Arg. Nit.	Paroxyms of cramps in esophagus, which feels spasmodically closed, producing after a meal.
Bryonia	Pressive, sticking pains and painful sensation of contraction, especially in lower portion, with inability to swallow.
Cactus Grand	Inflammatory or spasmodic state of the tissues of esophagus, with vomiting of all food before it reaches the stomach; constriction at throat, with full throbbing carotids.
Calc. Carb.	Organic stricture or spasmodic contraction and narrowness of esophagus, violent stiching in upper part of esophagus when not swallowing; sensation of rawness and soreness in entire esophagus, as if food had lodged there; cannot eat enough, food will not go down.
Cantharis	Difficult deglution with **NOCTURNL REGURGATION**; burning sensation in throt, which feels as if it were on fire; thirst, with aversion to all fluids.
Carbolic acid	Spasmodic and painful contraction of esophagus with inability to swallow; soreness of throat on empty deglution; choking feeling in throat, with disposition to hawk up phlegm.
Carbo veg	Sensation as if esophagus and pharynx were contracted and drawn together; NO PAIN, BUT FOOD IS NOT EASILY SWALLOWED; feeling of coldness in throat.
Crotalus	Deglution of any solid substance impossible (Bapt.); soup must be strained to remove all meat fibres and solid particles; nervous sore throt, PAIN OUT OF ALL PROPORTION TO THE VISIBLE TROUBLE (Lach); fauces dry; grat irritability and sensitiveness to dry and cold air.
Colchicum	Dysphagia, pain throt, larynx and muscles of neck; constriction in esophagus, with accumulation of mucus in throat, which comes involuntarily into mouth or is hawked.
Hepar	Sensation as if a fishbone or splinter were sticking in throat; sensation of a plug in throat, which feels dry.

Hyoscyamus	SPASMODIC CONTRACTION AFTER A PREVIOUS INJURY OF ESOPHAGUS; solids and warm food can be swallowed best; fluids cause spasm in throat, stop breathing and talking; hiccough, nausea, spasmodic cough and stiffness of muscles of neck.
Hydrocyanic acid	Spasm in pharynx and esophagus, with heat, inflammation and inability to swallow.
Ignatia	Dificulty in swallowing solids; sensation of lump in throat when swallowing, strangulating sensation in the middle of fauces as if a large lump had lodged in throat, hysterical patients.
Iodium	Inflammation and ulceration of esophagus; pain < by pressure; deglution extdremely painful and difficult; swelling of glands of neck; salivation; foetor oris.
Kali bich	Burning sensation of pharynx to stomach; pain and feeling as if something remained in esophagus after swallowing solid.
Kali carb	Food lodges in esophagus and causes gagging and vomiting; difficult swallowing small particles of food easily get into windpipe; stinging pains; great sensitiveness of esophagus, < after and drink, ONLY TEPID NOURISHMENT AGREES.
Lachesis	Sensation as if a button or crumb had lodged in throat; gagging and smothering when attempting to swallow, as if food had gone the wrong way, fluids return through nose; can swallow solids more easily than liquids; spasms rouse from sleep or develop as he awakes.
Laurocerasus	Spasmodic contraction of throat and esophagus with dysphagia; dull pain in throat with accumulation of tenacious mucus.
Lycopodium	Feeling of contraction in throat preventing deglusion; food and drink regurgitate through nose.

Continued...

AILMENTS OF OESOPHAGUS – Remedies	
Lyssin	(Hypochondrium) –Periodical spasms of esophagus; continual painful inclination to swallow without being able to do it; constriction most severe when trying to drink water, which causes burning and stinging pain in throat, cough and retching, which force the fluid from his mouth; difficult speech, palatic letters cannot be prounounced or only with difficulty.
Merc.sol	Dysphagia he has to press hard to get something down, aching pains in esophagus, spasmodic difficulty of swallowing, with danger of suffocation, liquids are ejected through nose.
Mezereum	Violent burning and soreness in upper part of esophagus; swallowing painful and difficult, especially after abuse of mercury.
Naja tripudians	Spasmodic stricture of esophagus, hardly anything can pass into the stiomach; laryngismus, from SPINAL IRRITATION AFFECTING NUCHA.
Nat. Mur.	Only fluids can be swallowed, solids when they reach a certain point are violently ejected, with gagging and attacks suffocation; hawking up of phlegm in the morning; constipation.
Nitric acid	Violent pain during deglution, can swallow only liquids; while eating, small pieces of food are forced into choanae.A
Oxalic acid	MORNING DISPHAGIA, with burning in throat and esophagus, with sour eructations and hawking up of thick phlegm.
Phosphorous	SPASMODIC STRICTURE OF ESOPHAGUS AT ITS CARDIAC END, regurgitation of all food, weak and empty feeling across abdomen, with occasional shooting pains; food reaches cardia and is at once rejected; great nervous irritability.

Plumbum	Fluids can be swallowed dasily, but solids come back into mouth; burning in esophagus and stomach some more hours after eating; spasmodic constriction with a sensation of a plug in throat, < when trying to swallow, sith great urging to do it; spasmodic dyspnoea; constipation, emaciation, debility.
Pulsatilla	Sensation on swallowing as if a back part of throat were narrower than usual or closed by swelling; sensation as if pharynx were swollen, difficulty of swallowing as if from paralysis of the muscles of deglution; choking in pharynx as from swallowing too large a morsel.
Rhus Tox	Solids are swallowed with difficulty owing to a feeling of contraction in esophagus, burning and soreness in throat.
Scilicea	Dysphagia, food passes slowly into stomach, no inflammation, rather more of a PARETIC STATE; throat feels as if filled up; frequent cough brings up white, frothy, saltish mucus, < towards evening.
Spigelia	Constricting pain constant and severe, passing through just to the back below the inferior angle of the right scapula (Laur.)., < from any attempt to swallow liquids or solid food, with vomiting; > by sucking small pieces of rice.
Stramonium	Violent constriction of throat, deglutition almost impossible, terrible spasms of throat when attempting to swallow.
Veratrum vir	Spasm of esophagus, with or without rising of frothy, blood mucus, constant inclination to swallow, dryness hiccough, nausea and vomiting.
Veratrum Alb.	SPASMS FOLLOWED BY PARALYSIS: nearly all food or drink taken is thrown up, attended by a sufficient sensation, with redness and heat in fac; often result of excitement and emotions.
Zincum met	Sensation of constriction and spasm of esophagus; small yellow ulcers on the inside of cheeks and in the throat; metallic or salty taste; formication of the skin.

Continued...

AILMENTS OF STOMOCH

ANATOMY:

This is a saccular dilatation of the digestive tract which is continuous with the esophagus above and with the duodenum below. It occupies a position on the left side of the abdomen, below the diaphragm and to the left of the liver. It is about twelve inches in length and four inches wide. Its long axis is obliquely from above, behind and to the left, downward, forward and to the right. It is wholly covered with peritoneum.

By reason of its loose peritoneal connection, it is one of the most movable of the abdominal organs. The cardiac end is the most fixed point, it is posterior to the seventh costal cartilage and one inch to the left of the sternum. The fundus rises behind and above the apex of the heart to the level of the sixth costochondral articulation. The location of the pylorus is not constant, it is usually one inch to the right of the median line and two inches below ensiform cartilage. The upper border is indicated by a short curve with its concavity upwards connecting with the cardiac and pylorus orifices. The greater curvature crosses the median line of the abdomen, midway between the ensiform cartilage and the umbilicus.

DYSPEPSIA:

Indigestion – Often a symptom of other diseases and characterised by vague abdominal discomfort, a sense of fullness after eating, eructation, nausea vomiting and loss of appetite. irregular eating habits, stress both of mental/physical, sleepless nights, consuming food exposed to open and unhealthy atmosphere, old and preserved food items even seems to be stored in the protective environments as is thought, especially non-veg items.

Needless to Submit that ediction to excessive alchohol consumption is the route cause for many of the health complaints. The pity is knowingly, most of them still continue the same.

DYSPEPSIA REMEDIES	
Abies Nigra	Total loss of appetite in the morning, craving for food at noon, and exceedingly hungry and wakeful at night; oain after a hearty meal, but abstinence from any particular food does not relieve the dyspepsia; belching and acid eructations, frequent vomiting, SENSATION AS IF SOME INDIGESTIBLE SUBSTANCE HAD STUCK IN THE CARDIAC END OF THE STOMACH (Lact.ac.); sensation as if all food lodged under upper end of stomach); continual distressing constriction just above the pit stomach, as if everything were knotted up, as if a hard lump of undigested food remained there, < whenever his vital energy is below par; hypochondriasis; constipation.
Aesculus Hip	HAEMORRHOIDAL patients, heartburn, waterbrash, empty eructations; burning pain in stomach after eating, lasting from one meal to another; nausea, vomiting; empty lasting from one meal to another; nausea, vomituration, or vomiting; empty eructations or bringing up thick phlegm; PRICKING IN HEPATIC REGION, with pains between shoulders and whole length of spine, bloatedness of abdomen; colic around navel, and incisive pain around navel; incessant to, desire to defaecate, provoked by pressure behind, with pruritus and sensation of ulceration of anus; bilious temperament, lassitude, confused of ideas; hypochondriasis.
Aethusa cyn	Violent vomiting of a frothy white substance, REGURGITATION OF FOOD AN HOUR OR SO AFTER EATING, or painful contraction of stiomach of such severity as to prevent vomiting; tearing, rending pains in pit of stomach, extending to esophagus; soreness and painfulness in both hypochondria; weakness and drowsiness, speech impeded, slow, breath short, interrupted by hiccough, pustules in throat, making patient nearly frantic, with burning in throat and dysphagia, sensation as if stomach were turned upside down, with burning feeling in chest.

Continued...

Abrotanum	CHLOROSIS. Disturbed digestion; weak, sinking feeling in bowels, food passes undigested; distended abdomen; great weakness and prostration; gnawing hunger, craves bread boiled in milk.
Agaricus musc	Epigastric pain, commencing to be felt about t here hours after eating, and daily renewing itself about the same time after a meal; burning, changing to a sensation of deep pressure, with nausea, vomiting and feeling of obstruction in throat; stitches in hypochondria and around navel; boborgmi, colic, constipation, during the paroxysm, convulsive motions of face and extremities, lips cyanosed; nervous persons, vertigo, with pale face and tendency to fall forward, nearly amaurotic weakness, with muscae volitantes; very drowsy after meals.
Allium sativum	Long-standing dyspepsia, especially in old fleshy people whose bowels are disturbed by the slightest deviation from the regular diet; copious flow of saliva after eating; belching or heartburn after every change of diet, weight in epigastrium immediately after a meal; cough, which seems to come from the stomach, dry cough after eating, GLUTTONY, COMPLAINTS OF THOSE WHO EAT TO EXCESS, pressure as from a stone in stomach, > by bending and pressure with hands.
Alertis far.	DYSPEPSIA FROM GENERAL DEBILITY; nausea, disgust for all food, the least food causes distress in stomach, frequent attacks of fainting, with vertigo, slow digestion, flatulence, constipation, sleepiness.
Alumen	Sinking sensation at epigastrium,< after eating; nervous exhaustion at the pit stomach, sensation of construction; cold sweat.
Allium Sativa	Long-standing dyspepsia, especially in old fleshy people whose bowels are disturbed by the slightest deviation from the regular diet, copious flow of saliva after eating; belching or heartburn after every change of diet; weight in epigastrium immediately after a meal; cough, which seems to come from the stomach, dry cough after eating, GLUTTONY, COMPLAINTS OF THOSE WHO EAT TO EXCESS; pressure as from a stone in stomach, > by bending and pressure with hands.

Alsotinia constr	ATONIC DYSPEPSIA, with loss of appetite, great debility and prostration, when recovering from severe acute affections or from malaria (compare Chin).
Alumina	DRYNESS, hence deficiency of gastric juice in stomach; irregular or excessive appetite, derangement of stomach and esophagus, so that even small portions of food are swallowed with difficulty; tingling itching at tongue loss of taste, heartburn, potatoes disagree, acrid, salty taste of all food; saliva salty, mouth feels dry; aversion to meat and craving for indigestible things, chronic indurated engorgement of glands, STUBBORN CONSTIPATION FROM INERTIA AND DRYNESS OF RECTUM; PRURITUS ANI.
Ambra	Sour eructations, aching in a small spot on right side of abdomen, in hepatic region, sensation of as a spoiled stomach and regurgitation of acid substances, as high up as the larynx, like heartburn, distension of stomach after every meal; incarcerated flatus; flatulent colic after midnight; frequent tenesmus, but n stool, with considerable anxiety; wants nobody around her, she must lie down on account of giddiness and sensation of weakness of stomach, < from warm drinks, especially warm milk; uneasy sleep, must get up; MENTAL WORRY.
Ammon. Carb	Pressure in stomach after eating and at night, the clothes feel oppressive; burning and heat in stomach, vomits all his food, afterwards sour taste in mouth continual thirst, no appétit e, except for bread and cold food < from warm food; cannot eat dinner without drinking; inclination to stretch limbs. Suitable to old women, who lead a sedentary life.
Amm. Mur	Lymphatic subjects without energy; ALL MUCOUS SECRETIONS AND RETAINED; bitter eructations, thirst for acids; REGURGITATION OF FOOD, hawking up sour mucus; nausea after ameal;heat andfulness in stomach; epigastric pain sets immediately after eating; heaviness of liver, bloatedness of abdomen, stools soft, glairy, or hard followed by tenesmus, and always covered covered with mucus; burning and smarting of anus after stool; lassitude increased by least exercise; no sleep after 3 AM constipation alternating diarrhoea.

Continued...

DYSPEPSIA REMEDIES	
Anacardium	FLATULENT DYSPEPSIA. PROSTRTION OF NERVOUS SYSTEM AND FUNCTIONAL LANGUOR OF STOMACH; often from excessive mental labor, exhaustion of nerve force, hence CONSTANT DESIRE TO EAT, which gives ease momentarily, but the hunger is never assuaged. And pain and distress may be again relieved by eating; he has to get up at night to eat something; flatulence from emptiness; tasteless or sour eructations.
Angustura Vera	PARTICULAR AVERSION TO MEAT AND GREAT LONGING FOR COFFEE; desires one thing or another and is disgusted with everything brought to her, bitter taste in mouth; bread tastes sour; nilious eructations andloss of appetite, often slight for stool. Craves warm drinks (Cascar, Cedr. Hyper.).
Antim. Crud.	Overloading the stomach and GASTRIC DERANGEMENT IN CHILDREN, WOMEN AND OLD PEOPLE; thickly quoted tongue, with anorexia, slow digestion and and foetid eructations, often followed by diarrhoea, particularly after acid wines or new beer; habitual sensation in stomach as if overloaded, excessive crossness, even hypochondriasis with suicidal tendencies; dryness of mouth with great thirst. < at night, constipation alternating with diarrhoea; helminthiasis, caused by overeating, hot weather, bathing, during measles, metastasis of gout and rheumatism.
Arg Nitricum	NERVOUS DYSPEPSIA; sharp stinging pains soon after taking food, with copious tasteless eructations, the stomach seems as if it would burst with wind, with great desire to belch, which is accomplished with difficulty, when the air rushes out with great violence, or vomiting of stringy, glairy mucus; after taking any fluid, it appears asifit were running straight through the intestinal canal, without stopping; loud rumbling in bowels; time seems to pass very slowly; moral and nervous disturbance, especially after dinner; < from anything cold, from candy, sugar, or sweet meats child cries with pain during eructation.

Arnica	After a meal sensation of impending apoplectic congestion of brain, with throbbing headache and drowsiness; sensation of lassitude and of fatigue; restlessness and agitation after a meal, burning heat in pit of stomach; frequent eructations, smelling of sulphuretted hydrogen, especially in the morning; bad taste when waking up; sour taste constantly in mouth, all that he eats tastes sour; thick brown tongue, complete loss of appetite; after eating, nausea vomiting; fullness of stomach and pressure as from a stone; cramps, stitches, burning; tendency to diarrhoea or lienteria; heat in head and coldness of other parts of body; fullness in epigatrium, with flatulence and distension of abdomen after a meal; feeling of indolence in the extremities, restlessness and disturbed sleep, cannot fin d a soft place or an easy position to sleep, dullness of head, especially forehead, and over the eyes, obscurity of sight, especially when moving head or walking; furunculosis.
Arsenicum	Dyspepsia, with heartburn, and belching up acid burning fluid, which seems to excoriate the throat; red and irritated tongue, which feels heated and rough to patient, as if scalded; burning heat in stomach and abdomen; epigastric swelling, with painfulness to pressure and even to contact to contact; sensation as if stomach were full of water, nausea, vomiting, and diarrhoea especially after drinking cold or acidulated water; RELIEF FROM HOT DRINKS; sensation of emptiness in stomach, so that he wants food, and still does not feel like eating when set before him; disgust for animal food; sensation of faintness, excessive sudden weakness, cold, extremities, cold skin. Dyspepsia from immoderate use of ice, vinegar, acid, or fermented liquors from abuse of tobacco, from ice-cream or oce-water in hot weather.

Continued...

Asafoetida	Enormous meterorismus of stomach, and great difficulty of bringing up wind (Arg.nit.); rancid eructations, flatus passing upword, none down, profuse salivation with greasy taste; burning in stomach and esophagus; pulsations in pit of stomach, with faint feeling; pressing, cutting-stitching, pains in spells, not regular; great disgust for food, appetite for wine; watery offensive diarrhoea or obstinate constipation; physical and mental over sensitiveness, hysteria.
Arum met.	Hypochondrias, with thoughts of suicide; immoderate apetite and thirst (Anac.), with qualmishness in stomach; relishes his meal, but appetite not appeased; aversion to meat, wants milk, wine, coffee, burning and pressure in stomach with hot risings, pressure in hypochondria as from flatulence, worse afer food, drink and motion, eructations of gas relieve attacks of palpitation; piles.
Baptisia	Great sinking at the epigastrium, with frequent fainting; irritation of stomach; showing itself by violent pains at short intervals over the whole cardiac region, with anguish and a burning sensation, TONGUE BROWN IN CENTRE AND RED AT EDGES, nausea, with want of appetite and constant desire for water; frequent small diarrhoeic stools, but excessively foetid; pain in liver. Excessive prostration of strength, after typhoid fever, with general debility, trembling, weak, soft pulse, atony of all functions and undefinable malaise.
Baryta carb	Nause early in the morning; sourish eructations daily a few hours after dinner; pain and pressure at the stomach as from stone; relieved by eructations; even when fasting a soreness is felt at the stomach; gnawing pains in stomach not aggravated by pressure; the passage of food into the stomach is painful, as if it passed over a sore spot; sensation of weakness in stomach, disappearing after eating. Dyspepsia developed due to the habit of masturbation.

Belladonna	Face flushed or very pale; eyes red, putrid taste in fauces, also while eating and drinking, although food tastes natural; nausea in throat, painless throbbing and beating in pit of stomach, feeling of emptiness in stomach, hard pressure in stomach after eating.
Berberies vul.	Offenstive metallic odor from mouth; mouth fauces dry and sticky, especially in the morning, relieved by eating, before dinner chilliness, after eating solids belching for hours and soreness, continuing all night; heartburn; pressure in stomach as if it would burst, pit of stomach puffed up (Calc.) great thirst or aversion to drink, <after alcoholic drink.
Bismuth	Headache alternating with or attended by gastralgia. Sweetish and metallic taste; copious and continuous secretion of a thick saliva, brown and of a metallic taste; sensation of excoriation in mouth; swelling and sensitiveness of gums; burning heat in throat, great thirst for cold beverages; HE VOMITS THE SMALLEST QUANTITY OF WATER, ALTHOUGH THE STOMCH RETAINS EVERYTHING ELSE; COUGH WHEN STOMACH IS EMPTY; soon after eating, burning and pressure in stomach, circumscribed on a narrow point and forcing patient to bend backward; nausea; eructations of a bad odour; vomituration and vomiting; loud boborgmi and flatulency; malaise in lower abdomen; constipation, or watery, foul-smelling diarhhoea, urine abundant and limpid. Distress extends from stomach through to spine, with burning in spine opposite epigastrium.
Bovista	Nausea in the morning, vomiting of a watery fluid, relieved by eating breakfast, SENSATION OF A LUMP OF ICE IN THE STOMACH; pressure and fulness in pit of stomach; tension in temples, mental anguish.

Continued...

Bryonia	DYSPEPTIC AILMENTS DURING SUMMER HEAT, especially moist heat (Ant.crud) acute, recent cases, caused by high living, or where fruits produce painful bloating of stomach; dry mouth and throat, yellow coat of tongue, aphthae, empty or bitter belching; everything tastes bitter, hence desire for stimulants; GREAT SENSITIVENESS OF EPIGASTRIUM TO TOUCH; pressure of clothing produces pain, but not always oppression o breathing; nausea and faintness on rising from a recumbent position; distension in intestines rather than in stomach; after a meal, sensation of fullness in stomach or as if a stone lat there, < moving; water-brash; icteric tint of the skin, and skin and eyes; congestive headaches; obstinate constipation, differing from Nux.vom. by the absence of desire, without result; intolerance of vegetable food, <in summer.
Caladium	Throbbing and beating in epigastrium, with debility and languor, obliging the patient to lie down, and fainting sensation when getting up; FLUTTERING AS FROM A BIRD in the stomach causes nausea; burning in stomach not relieved by drink, frequent eructations of very little wind, as if he stomach were full of dry food, acrid sour vomit, making teeth feel too long; aversion tp cold drinks; WANTS ONLY WARM BEVERAGES (Ars.), restless and starting in sleep.
Capscicum	DIPSOMANIA: morning vomiting, sinking at stomach; stomach cold or burning in it; dyspepsia from torpor, particularly in old people; flatulence and wind colic; hearatburn, waterbrash; food tastes sour, bitter while eating, worse afterwards, water causes shuddering; purging, tenemus, and thin stools, anxiety and fear of dying, peevish, irritable, angry; foul breath; haemmorhoids, lack of reaction, VERY OFFENSIVE BREATH WHEN COUGHING.

DYSPEPSIA REMEDIES	
Carbo veg.	PATIENT PHYSICALLY BELOW PAR; dyspepsia after abuse of mercury, or from too high living (Nux.vom) EXCESSIVE FLATULENCY WITH TENDENCY TO DIAHRRHOEA, dyspeptic sufferings come on most severly after breakfast; sensation as if he would burest open after eating or drinking; nausea every morning from 10 until 11, gastric troubles after drinking wine or ardent spirits to excess; sensation of trembling and weight in athe stomach, the thought of taking food causes nausea and disgust, violent spasmodic contraction in epigastric region, better by fright, chagrin, cold or taking food; GASTRALGIA OF NURSING WOMEN, the whole mouth seems bitter, bitter eructations; milk is insupportable, turns sour; repugnance to meat and especially to fat, to fish, oysters, vinegar; hiccough heaviness and dullness of head; cannot bear any pressure around the waist; sensation of pressure and fullness along the edges of the false ribs in both hypochondria, the diaphragm being pushed out of its place by the accumulated gas, with painful respiration, vertigo and faint ness during and after meals; CHRONI DYSPEPSIA OF OLD PEOPLE; incarcerated flatulence, < leaning back with a pillow under part complained of.
Carduus mar:	GASTRIC AILMENTS FROM ABUSE OF ALCHOLIC DRINKS AND ESPECIALLY OF BEER, gastric catarrah with loss of appetite, frequent eructations, flatulency; burning in stomach, as from acidity, bitter taste, intense nausea, painful retching and vomiting of sour, greenish fluid; pressure in stomach with eructations of air, at night on awakening, lasting all day, hepatic region sensitive to pressure, pasty diarrhoea. "Bergucht," phthisis of miners, a complex of symptoms of stomach, spleen and kidneys with insomnia, inappetency, mental irritability, languor and general weakness.

Continued...

Cedran	Bitter eructations before rising in the morning, with a dull pain in temples; sensation of a stone in stomach, of heat and fullness in stomach; distension and disposition to nausea, <by rest,> by walking and eating; great sensitiveness of praecordial region; pulse small and hard, dryness of mouth and fauces, depressed spirit and restlessness, RELIEVED BY FOOD AND DRINK.
Chelidoneum	Tongue dry and white, sometimes streaky, of narrow and pointed shape; great longing for wine, does not cause congestion or heat in head as formerly; aching gnawing pain in stomach, with a sense of constriction, aggravated by pressure, but RELIEVED BY EATING or during the early hour of digestion; great desire for milk, which when drinking it; PREFERENCE FOR HOT DRINKS AND FOR HOT FOOD; gurgling in abdomen, colic, retraction of navel, with nausea, incisive intentional pains, constipation; icterus; morose disposition; constant pain under lower inner angle of right scapula, extending up into chest and down to liver.
Chinium Sulph	EXCESSIVE REPUGNANCE TO ALL FOOD; swelling and sensitiveness of epigasgrium; oppression after eating, nausea, desire to sleep, visceral obstructions, especial engorgement of spleen; loss of all energy; somnolence in day time.

DYSPEPSIA REMEDIES	
China	Dyspepsea from loss of animal fluids, from noxious miasmata; face pale or swallow, tongue foul, white or yellow, CONTINUAL SENSATION OF SATIETY, of coldness in stomach, and desire for pungent, spiced, sour, refreshing things, for coffee-beans and for stimulants; extreme slowness of digestion; pressure and cramps of stomach after eating; malaise, drowsiness, fullness, distension; eructations, tasting after the food, and even vomiting the ingesta; desire to lie down; sense of sinking at the epigastrium, relieved by eating, but speedily retuning; aggravation from fariness food; obstructed respiration; liquid lienteric stools immediately after eating; urine dark-coloured and heavy; sleep frequently disturbed; ill-humor and indisposition to do anything; fruit induce diarrhoea with abdominal fermentation, but little or no relief; from belching; DIARRHOEA WITH GOOD, or even increasing appetite, especially after meals (Ant.crud., diarrhoea with total inappetency); aversion to fat, to warm food and drinks, which disagree with the stomach, < every other night.
Chionanthus	BILIOUS DYSPEPSIA; hypochondriasis, weant to be let alone, tongue of dirty, greenish-yellow or colour and very dry, though usual quantity of saliva; setting teeth on edge, stomach feels weak and empty,> by eating; foul flatus.
Cina	Desires many and different things; great hunger soon after eating; on drinking wine she shudders as though it were vinegar, hiccough; during sleep; gnawing sensation in stomach, as from hunger, pressure in stomach at night, causing restlessness, as from hunger; pressure in stomach at night, causing restlessness; diarrhoea after drinking; vomiting of mucus, with weak, hollow, empty feeling in head; grinding of teeth.

Continued...

Cocculus	Chronic dyspepsia, from abuse of stimulants or from too long studies; confused feeling in head after eating or drinking; nausea with vertigo and afflux of saliva; morning nausea and vomiting of food and mucus, especially at night, with sleeplessness, headache and constipation, absolute loss of appetite; burning in esophagus extending into fauces, with taste of sulphur in mouth; acid taste in mouth, with aversion to acids, after eating, pains of contusion, of pressure, of grinding and squeezing in the pit of stomach; lower extremities seem nearly paralyzed; EXTRME AVERSION TO FOOD, EVEN THE SMALL OF FOOD SICKENS, ALTHOUGH HE FEELS HUNGRY.
Collinsonia	Haemmorrhoidal dyspepsia and headache; tongue yellow along centre of base, with bitter taste; cramp like pains in stomach, with nausea; flatulence and spasms of stomach; chronic constipation, with much flatulence and haemorrhoids.
Conium	Violent paint in stomach always TWO OR THREE HOURS AFTER EATING, but also at night; better in knee-elbow position; violent vomiting of BLACK MASSES LIKE COFFEE-GROUNDS, sour and acrid; sour rising from stomach after eating; swelling in region of pylorus; pressing, burning, squeezing pain, extending from pit of stomach into the back and shoulders (Bism.); hypochondriasis.
Cornus circ	Nausea, with bitter taste an aversion to all kinds of food; empty feeling in stomach, with tasteless eructations; desire for sour drinks; smarting and burning in mouth, throat and stomach, with desire for stool; sensation of faintness in stomach and abdomen
Cuprum	Deathly feeling, with pain behind the ensiform cartilage; express ion of prostration in face; sweet or coppery taste; tongue dry and rough, papillae enlarged; loss of appetite; GREAT DESIRE FOR COOLING DRINKS; a swallow of cold water relieves cough and vomiting; hiccough; constant eructations, nausea and VOMITING WITH BRAIN AFFECTIONS, from suppression of menses; sensation as if clothing were lying too hard on pit of stomach.

Cyclamen	Complete inappetency, feeling of satiety after a few mouthfuls of food; great pain in pit of stomach, > after throwing up the food; disgust for meat; pork disagrees; aversion to coffee and desire for inedible things; sleepiness, hiccough during and after eating; rumbling in bowels; chlorosis, with great read of fresh air.
Cypripedium	Dyspepsia, the result of mental over-exertion, anxiety or grief.
Digitalis	After eating a weakness in stomach as if the stomach sinking away or as if life would vanish; deathly nausea, not > by vomiting; appetite for food, but as soon as he eats HE COMMENCES IT SPIT IT UP BY MOUTHFULS, SOURER THAN ANY VINEGAR; after stomach is emptied, terrible and uneasiness for one or two hours; discomfort after eating even a small quantity of light food; extreme lassitude and trembling; quick, intermitting or very slow pulse, bowels confined, urine dark and scanty, feeling of great or emptiness of stomach just before going to sleep; sleep uneasy and unrefreshing; surface and extremities cold and blue.
Dulcamra	Flat, soapy taste with loss of appetite; natural taste, with good appetite but soon satiated; frequent pinching and distension of abdomen; copious eructations with scraping in esophagus and heartburn; quamishness and nausea, vomiting of tenacious mucus with warm rising in esophagus in the morning; pressing pain in epigastrium, as from a blow, > on pressure; sensation of soreness in spinal cord and occiput; indigestion with chilliness; sensation of sorenbess in spinal cord and occiput; indigestion with chilliness,< every cool change of weather.
Elaps coral	STOMACH INTOLERANT OF ANYTHING COLD; fruits, ice-cream and ot her cold things like cold lumps of ice on the stomach and cause cold feeling in chest; acidity of stomach with nausea and faint feeling, > by lying on abdomen, desire for sweetened buttermilk; sudden pain in stomach as if she would sink down, < while sitting, > walking about.

Continued...

Eupatorium Perf	Insipid taste, disgust for food; desire for ice-cream, ANOREXIA OF DRUNKARDS; belching of tasteless wind, with a feeling of obstruction at the pit of stomach, shuddering proceeding from stomach; qualmishness from odours, smell of food, cooking, etc.
Fel bovis	Dry tongue, eructations; borborygmi in epigastrium and abdomen, flatulent dyspepsia, incomplete digestion of food, constipation of soft stool; when nearly done he can still press out some faecal lumps; DYSPEPSIA OF CONVALESCENTS FROM SEVERE ACUTE DISEASES (Kreos.)
Fel vulpis	Dyspepsia, based on lassitude of the whole intestinal canal, hence flatulency constipation, foul lienteric stools from decomposition of food.
Ferr. Met	Increase of the watery elements of the blood and decrease of solids; relaxation and debility after an excitation which might be mistaken for exuverance of life; unbearable taste of blood, of rotten eggs, loathing for sour things, of meat, which disagrees, of hot things (Calc.carb.) solid food is dry and insipid while masticating, appetite good and bad alternately, nausea, with headache, nightly diarrhoea; VOMITING IMMEDIATELY AFTER EATING; heavy pressure in pit of stomach after every meal; painless and involuntary diarrhoea, with undigested food, or constipation from intestinal atony. Wind dyspepsia.
Ferrum Phos	Anorexia, aversion to milk,< from meat and sour things; nausea and vomiting after eating; vomited matter so sour that it sets teeth on edge, hammering pains in forehead and temples; chronic diarrhoea or costiveness; sleep restless and dreamy, great depression in the morning.

Fluoric acid	Chronic irritation of mucous membranes; disagreeable mood, dull heavy headache; hunger and thirst, especially for wine; complaints worse from sweets, bilious vomiting after slight errors in diet, with increased alvine discharges, preceded by tormina, feeling of weight in stomach between meals; fullness and pressure in epigastrium; bilious diarrhoea soon after drinking, especially warm drinks.
Graphites	Salty, sour foul taste in mouth aversion to food, especially to meat and salt food; unpleasant sensation before eating; during a meal immediate effects, especially abdominal distension, borborygmi, after eating burning, sticking, cramps, singultus, nausea, must loosen the clothing; rotten odour from mouth and gums, especially after rising, lessened by washing out the mouth, canine hunger with acidity of stomach or none with fullness of stomach; SWEET THINGS ARE DISGUSTING AND NAUSEOUS; HOT THINGS DISAGREE; rancid heartburn, particularly after eating; excessive discharge of foul flatus downward; obstinate constipation with very hard stools, expelled only after great efforts, or pappy, half-digested, brown stool of a most atrocious odour, large protruding haemorrhoidal tumours; humid or crusty eruptions; unhealthy rough and harsh skin; breath smells like urine; flabby obesity; < mornings and from cold; suffocative spells arousing from sleep, must jump out of bed and eat something.
Gratiola	Great distension of abdomen after meals; pressure at the pit of stomach as from a stone rolling from side to side with cramp-like drawing which mounts into the chest, frequent urging to eructate and to vomit; great lassitude and somnolence after meals; APPETITE FOR NOTHING BUT BREAD; aversion to smoking; cold feeling in stomach, as if full of water; cramps in stomach.

Continued...

Helonias	Great prostration of nervous system, anaemia, pulse small and feeble, paleness and icteric colour of skin; loss of appetite, bitter taste; constricting, pressing pain in stomach; empty eructations, vomiting, borborgmi and sensation as if diarrhoea would set in, but stools are regular; tongue red at tip and borders, white in centre, albuminuria, diabetes, sorrowfulness and melancholy; patient excitable and wishes to be let alone, renal and uterine troubles.
Hep. Sulph	ATONIC DYSPEPSIA. Hunger, a gnawing, empty feeling in stomach during forenoon, relieved by eating, but food causes feeling of fullness, he cannot bear any pressure upon epigastrium; desire for acid food and drinks, for condiments and wine; flatulence, but without much soreness, burning sensation in scrubiculo cordis; considerable epigastric swelling, even after eating but little; LIABILITY TO DERANGEMENT OF STOMACH IN SPITE OF THE MOST CAREFUL DIET; foetid eructtions, with sensation of burning in athroat, nausea mornings, perhaps with sour, bilious or slimy vomiting; accumulation of mucous in throat, aversion to fat; great thirst, constipationwiath infectual urging to stool, faeces not being hard, slightly coloure or white diarrhoea. Antidotes mercurial abuse.
Hydrastis	ATONIC DYPEPSIA; cancerous diathesis. Great lassitude, debility, exhaustion, obstinate constipation, and its attendant dull headache in the forehead, urging to urinate, and sensation as if bowels would move, but only wind passes, large, flabby, slim-looking tongue, sour eructations; cannot digest bread and vegetables, empty, ACHING, GONE FEELING IN STOMACH, aggravated by eating, WEAKNESS OF DIGESTION, WITH HEAVY, DULL, HEADACHE, aggravated by eating,, DULL, HEAD, THUMPING FULNESS OF CHEST AND DYSPNOEA, palpitation of heart, even light pressure of hand reveals strong pulsations in pit of stomach, faintings from exhaustion;

	eructations of a bitter fluid, pyrosis; burning pains in umbilical region, with stitches in epigastrium extending to testicles, appearing after tool and accompanied by great weaknes, haemorrhoids; sympathetic sore throat;chronic mucous discharges; like Nux.v. after abuse of drugs.
Hydrocyanic acid	Vomiting, acidity, waterbrash (pancreatic digestion at fault) pain immediately above the navel, two or three hours after eating, with sensitivenes of pressure at that spot,, it feels as if some resisting body lay there; vomiting, especially in the evening and at night, bilious or of the ingesta; burning pain above the navel, extending upward to esophagus; loss of appetite; colicky attacks; white-coated tongue, emaciation; < evenings and at night; dyspepsia upon chronic inflammation of tomach and bowels.
Ignatia	DYSPEPSIA WITH GREAT NERVOUS PROSTRATION, caused by mental depression; excessive sweat during a meal; copious salivation; feeling of weakness and sinking at the epigastrium,> momentarily by eating but soon returning. Mouth full of mucous, taste flat; food has a bitter. repulsative taste; fanciful aversion to special articles of food, or craving for a particular article, and after a small portion has been enjoyed, sudden and great aversion to it; frequent regurgitation of food and bitter liquid; EMPTY REETCHING RELIEVED BY EATING; painful bloating after a meal, with hiccough after eating and drinking; great emptiness with qualmishness and weakness in region of stomach, patient vomits at night the food taken in the evening, with flat taste in mouth; periodical paroxysms of cramps in stomach, stitching and lancinating in the sides abdomen; flatulent colic, especially at night, hard stools,he tries often, but in vain to defaecate, prolapsus recti while defaecting, pruritis and tingling in ano; difficult respiration as if the chest were compressed; at night palpitations; aversion to tobacco, meat warm food and spirituous drinks.

Continued...

DYSPEPSIA REMEDIES	
Iodium	Fasting causes pain in chest and heartburn after heavy food; aching pain in forehead, followed by canine hunger, and this by discharge of thin faeces; tension in stomach and bowels, renewed by eating; intense thirst,< from milk; heaches after dinner; large, full pulse and cerebral congestoioms.
Ipecacuanha	Gastric symptoms from and after indulgence in rich mixwed food, as pastry, fruits, sweets, ice-cream, bursting heaedache with deathly nausea, tongue clean or only slightly coated, stools green, yellow, liquid and covered with mucus and blood, stomach feels relaxed, as if hanging down, attacks of clutching pains, going from left to right, as from a hand, each finger seemingly pressing sharply into intestines,> during rest, < from motion.
Iris vers	Nausea and vomiting of watery and extremely sour fluid, especially during early morning, CONSTANT AND PROFUSE FLOW OR ROPY SALIVA, hanging in a string from the mouth to the vessel on the floor; great burning distress in epigastrium; shocks of pain from umbilical region up to epigastrium, before each spell of vomiting or purging, vomiting of food an hour after eating, of bile with great heat and sweat, yellow, watery, corrosive stool, with burning in rectum and anus after it.
Kali bichrom	ALTERNATION OF GASTRIC CATARRAH WITH RHEMATISM; supra-orbital neuralgia induced by gastric derangement; obscuration of sight followed by headache, < from light or noise, blindness diminishing as the headache increases, patient unable to digest any starchy food, immediately during or after a meal a sensation as if digestion were impeded and the food rested in stomach like a heavy weight (not a pain); patient wakes at night with great uneasiness in stomach and **soreness and tenderness in a small spot to the left of the xiphoid process**; feeling of sinking in stomach before breakfast;

	feeling of emptiness in stomach, though he has no appetite and feels worse after eating, hot risings from stomach, especially after taking oily food, champagne, beer or malt liquors, flatulency, dislike to water, which derange the stomach, < at night after lying down, with sour eructations; fibrid-red complexion, blotchy appearance and heavy skin; mucous membrane of digestive and respiratory organs simultaneously affected, with excessive secretion of both. CHRONIC EFFECTS OF EXCESSIVE INDULGENCE IN BEER AND ALE.
Kali brom	Anorexia, foul breath, white tongue, involving the edges as well as the dorsum, and not necessarily furred, grant languor; violent headache, loathing vomitutration or vomiting of mucus, with saltish taste in mouth; vomiting of drunkards after a debauch; troublesome pressure at stomach after dinner.
Kali Mur	Violent hunger between regular periods of eating,> after drinking water; white or grayish coating of tongue; pain or heavy feeling in hepatic region; fatty food disagree; portal congestion; gagging andgulping up white mucus; vomiting of slime or blood.

Continued...

DYSPEPSIA REMEDIES	
Kali carb	DYSPEPSIA OF AGED PERSONS rather inclined to obesity, or after great loss of vitality; repugnance to all food, constant chilliness, cold hands and feet, no perspiration however, great the heat is; face pale, eyes sunken, oedema of upper eyelid, dryness of mouth, dull taste, tongue yellowish-white; lips dry, thirst, great desire for sugar and sweets, for acids; aversion to rye bread, epigastrium swollen, hard, sensitive to touch; painful sensation of emptiness in stomach, and, after eating ever so little, great feeling of fullness and pressure, which soon gives way to a sensation of goneness accompanied by bloatedness and eructations, especially after soup and coffee; burning after eating ever so little, great feeling fullness and pressure, which soon gives way to a sensation of goneness accompanied by bloateness and eructations, especially after soup and coffee; burning after eating, and rising from stomach to throat, great pain in the cul-de-sac and extremities; pulsation in epigastrium; nausea, eructationss, vomiting of food and mucus; bloatedness of abdomen, which is painful to touch; constipation as from inertia of rectum; stools dry, rare, difficult to discharge, feels badly before stool, bloody haemorrhoids; frequent desire to urinate during night; pale-red, muddy urine passes slowly and burns; RIGHT EAR HOT, LEFT EAR PALE AND COLD; vertigo from least motion,especially riding in carriage; respiration difficult, anxious; sleepiness or restless sleep after 3 a.m. grat irritability and sadness.
Kreosotom	DEEP AND LASTING DISGUST FOR FOOD IN CONVALESCENTS from severe dieases, as the least quantity of food or drink fatigues them equally; after several hours the food is thrown up undigested; great and constant nausea and inclination to vomit, but without actual sickness; cold feeling at the epigastrium internally, as if cold water or ice were there; tension over the stomach and scrobiculum; cannot bear tight clothing. Painful hard spots at or near the left of stomach; water tastes bitter, worse from cold, better from warm food; constipation, stool hard and expelled only after great effort;

	debility, weariness from a slight exertion, better after sleeping.
Lachesis	WEAK DIGESTION FROM VICIOUS HABITS; VOMITING OF DRUNKARDS; everything tastes sour, food becomes violently acid as soon as it reaches the stomach, great weakness of digestion with many eructations, scarecely any sort of food agrees, constant desire to swallow and when swallowing, sensation as if he had a foreign body in throat which cannot be moved upward or downward; stomach hard and distended, with flatulent colic; gnawing in the stomach relieved by eating, but returning in a few hours as soon as the stomach is empty, nausea vomiting of food, bile or mucus, especially after eating; immoderate desire for wine, craving for milk and oysters which often disagree, pale, sunken face, vertigo, constipation with hard and difficult stool at night; fruit and acids easily cause diarrhoea; cannot bear the pressure of clothing around the waist.
Leptandra	Nausea, with deathly faintness, upon rising in the night; painful distress in stomach, with rising of food, very sour; canine gunger; sharp cutting pains in the lower part of epigastrium and upper portion of umbilical region, weak sinking in pit of stomach; great distress in stomach and liver, worse from drinking water; stools black; tarry,bilious, undigested, followed by griping, but no straining.
Lithium carb	Pain in left temple, great lassitude and debility,gnawing in stomach the whole morning, going off after eating, but appetite is soon satisfied; after eating acidity and heaviness in stomach; great thirst without fever; fullness in pit of stomach, cannot endure the least pressure, he must loosen his clothing, diarrhoea after fruit and chocolate; the pain in head, which ceased while eating, returns, to be again relieved by eating. Constant desire to urinate, with some difficuly in urinating, and a press ing in cardiac region,> by urinating though violent tenesmus afterwards, < at night, pain in sacrum and lower limbs.

Continued...

Lobelia infl.	Sense of weakness and oppression of epigastrium and simultaneous oppress of chest, with or without heartburn, constant dyspnoea, <from slightest exertion, pain in forehead from one temple to other, sensation of a lump in pit of throat, impeding respiration and deglutition; no appetite, fullness and pressure in epigastrium < after eating; difficulty of breathing from faintness and sinking at the stomach; acidity, heartburn, lateritous urine. After each vomiting sweat all over, followed by sensation as if lots of needles were piercing the skin from within outward; faintness at pit of stomach from abuse of tea or tobacco.
Lycopodium	Atonic dyspepsia of weakly persons, INTESTINAL FLATULENT DYSPEPSIA (CARB.VEG. GASTRIC), from heavy farinaceous food, from fresh vegetables or leguminosea. CONSTANT SLEEPINESS, BUT SLEEP DOES NOT REFRESH; desire for food (which has its natural flavour) from a sensation of weakness in stomach but appetite is quickly satisfied on account of pressure on the stomach, as soon as he begins to eat; sour taste, and in the morning bitter taste, epigastric pain not increased by external pressure, eructations relieve the sense of repletion, but not increased by external pressure, eructations relieve the sense of repletion, but not the feeling of illness, empty and sour eructations, with sour taste; of everthing, even sweets, < from cold drinks,> from warm drinks, AS HOT AS MOUTH AND THROAT CAN BEAR THEM; incarcerated flatus, causing bloating and distension and asthamatic symptoms,with pains shooting across from right to left, < 4 to 8 p.m.: palpitation of heart during digestion; sensitiveness of gastric region to pressure only after a meal (Lach., all the time); CHRONIC CATARRAH OF STOMACH FROM ENLARGED LIVER, jaundiced or swallow complexion, with oedma pedum; grat mental depression; lithic acid gravel in urine; constipation or slow stool, the discharges always incomplete.

Magnesia carb.	ACID DYSPEPSIA. Extreme bloatedness of stomach, without eructations or flatulence, or with sour eructations and pyrosis after having eaten CABAGE, POTATOES AND OTHER GROSS FOOD; dryness of mouth burning in throat and palate; frequent rising of mucus in the throat, violent thirst for water, nausea and vertigo while eating, followed by retching and vomiting of a bitter salt water; constrictive pain in stomach.
Magneasia Mur	Continual rising of white froth into the mouth; eructations tasting like onions, fainting nausea succeeded by coldness and weakness of stomach; and gulping up of water, hunger, but knows not for what, followed by nausea; violent thirst towards morning; throbbing; eroding pains in stomach, going off after eating and coming on again at the end of digestion; stools in hard, large lumps, crumbling at the verge of the anus, knotty, like sheep's dung, exhaustion after sea-bathing.
Mancinella	Vertigo bitter taste, with burning and pricking in mouth; whole mouth and tongue covered with small vesicles; offensive breath; heat in pharynx and down esophagus, without thirst for cold water, but is prevented from drinking by the choking sensation rising from stomach; excessive nausea; SOUR GREASY VOMIT, with aversion to water; on the vomited matter floats a white mass like coagulated fat; sensation as of flames rising from stomach, or as if stomach grew together in a lump and then suddenly opened again, fullness in rectum, with a hollow feeling in stomach, diarrhoea in alternation with constipation.
Merc.sol.	Foul, sweetish or bitter taste, especially early in the morning; loss of appetite, or voracious, with speedy repletion after eating; aversion to solid food, wine or brandy, peculiar deadly faintness caused by pressure in epigastrium; eructations, heartburn, nausea, desire to vomit; painful sensitiveness, fullness, pressure, tension in gastric region; flatulence; constipation, often with ineffectual urging to stool and tenesmus; sadness, hypochondriasis, suspicious and vehement mood, patient cannot lie on right side.

Continued...

Merc. Cor.	REPUGNANCE TO HOT FOOD AND GREET DESIRE FOR COLD FOOD; putrid taste in morning, increased saliva, baad breath, bilious taint, the liver rises above the ribs; oppression after eating; distension and painful sensitiveness of stomach, eructations, nausea, tendency to diarrhoea, with tenesmus; copious excessive respiration, without relief.
Mezereum	CANINE HUNGER NOON AND EVENING; burning and uneasiness in stomach, relieved by eating; wants ham, fat, coffee and wine, beer tastes bitter and causes vomiting; abdomen distended by flatulence; the blood seems to leave her extremities and make her feel weak and giddy, with inability to speak, abundant foetid before stool, consisting of dark-brown. Hard balls.
Natrum sulph	Thick, tenacious white mucus constantly in the mouth, swelling up from the stomach; belching up mucus which is always foul and slimy; distension of and weight in the stomach with vomiting of bitter or sour mucus; great flatulence and cutting pains in abdomen, cannot bear clothing tight around waist; burning pinching in stomach and bowels, difficult breathing evening in bed; cough with all-gone empty, sensation in chest, no urging to stool, but difficult expulsion even of a soft stool, < in protracted damp, cloudy weather; diarrhoea every morning, after rising and moving about, accompanied by discharge of much foetid flatus.

DYSPEPSIA REMEDIES	
Nux moschata	Dyspepsia of hysterical women, given to sleepiness, fainating or laughing hysteria, with feeling as though the food formed itself fainting or laughing hysteria, with feeling as though the food formed itself into small hard lumps, with hard surfaces and angles, which produce soreness of stomach; dyspeptic symptoms come on at once, while patient is still at the table; she eats with appetite, but a few mouthfuls satisfy her; turuning in stomach with some nausea; mouth and throat dry, no thist, saliva like cotton, chalky taste, vomiting of digested food, with tough mucus of somewhat bitter or sour taste (Nux.v); immediately after eating or while person is still at table there is enormous abdominal distension with sensation as if food in the stomach had formed into hard lumps; heartburn; distended condition of stomach and abdomen, with sensation of warmth not only after a meal, but also from least contradiction, showing its nervous character; retrocession of gout to stomach, < from cool moisture, > by external warmth; syncope from nervous weakness.
Nux vomica	ATONY OF THE GANGLIONIC SYSTEM OF NERVES; first half of tongue clean, sometimes red and shining, but the posterior half is coated with a deep fur, food and drink have their normal taste, but immediately after eating ever so little, fullness and swelling of epigstgrium, which is sensitive to pressure, pyrosis, acid eructations, borborygmi, sqeezing around the waist, lassitude, nausea, with or without vomiting; head dull and painful, confusion of ideas; after a meal, pain in epigastrium, with sensation as if he had stones in tomach, pain in epigastrium, with sensation as if he had stones in stomach, pain limited to small spot, bitter, especially mornings, with little or no appetite, bread, acids, milk disagree, but all food aggravates, taste in the morning sour, bitter or putrid after raising mucus from throat; marked aggravation two hours after eating (duodenal digestion?); mental and physical over – impressionability; constipation with frequent and useless desire to defaecate, with sensation as if anus were closed. Gourmands et gourmets! Abuse of alcoholic drinks.

Continued...

Oleander	EXTREME DEBILITY OF DIGESSTIVE POWER; vomiting of food just as taken many hours after a meal, food has a weak, insipid taste, ravenous hunger, with trembling of hands, and hasty eating without appetite; violent empty eructatiion while eating; vomiting of food and bitter greenish water; after vomiting ravenous hunger and thirst; sudden sinking in pit of stonmach as if beats of heart were felt through whole thorax; lienteria, burning at anus before and after stool.
Pepsin	Dyspepsia of infants and convalescents, especially where they lost a great deal of blood and have been otherwise weakned; lienteria; pot-belliedness of children (Calc.c).
Petroleum	DYSPEPSIA ALWAYS RELLIEVED BY TAKING FOOD (Chel.):ATONIC DYSPEPSIA, with tendency tio diarrhoea and vomiting; pain and tenderness in epigastrium, occasional pysrosis; chilly cold abdomen; severe pains in stomach, radiating to chest, with sweat and nausea; aversion to meat, fat and to all warm, cooked food; violent thirst for beer, after eating, gastralgia better, but food causes giddiness, heat in face and cutting in abdomen; diarrhoea during day time, never at night, with colic before defaecation and hunger immediately after stool.

DYSPEPSIA REMEDIES	
Phosphorus	RUMINATION; acute and chronic dyspepsia, great weakness, cardiac anguish at night with nausea and a peculiar craving for, relieved by eating; very weak, empty, gone feeling felt in the whole abdominal cavity, often accompanied by a sensation of heat in back between shoulder-blades; burning in stomach, with desire for very cold water which relieves memomentarily, but is soon thrown up again as it gets warm in the stomach; dryness of throat at night, it fairly glistens; desire for cold food and drink, ice-cream; aversion to sweets and to meat; REGURGGITATION OF FOOD BY MOUTHFULS, WITHOUT NAUSEA; food scarcely swallowed come up again from spasm of esophagus at cardiac end, tympanitis, especially in caecum and colon tranversum; loud borborymi, tiring one out by their noise, momemntary relief by passing flatus; sensation of coldeness in abdomen, soft, watery, painless stools, beating of heart; congestion to head; hectic fever; night sweats.
Plantago	Frequent empty etuctations, sometimes with the taste of sulphur, heaviness of stomach even after a light meal; sensation of heat in the praecordia, with fullness in abdomen while walking in the fresh air, better when sitting down; faint and tremulous feeling, with nausea; slight appetite and speedy satiety, food tasteless; rumbling in abdomen after eating; loud and copious flatulency; diarrhoea with loose frequent stools and flatulence; haemorrhoids.
Podophylum	Changeable appetite; avidity for acids, putrid taste, foul breath, dryness of mouth and throat, tongue dry and white, after eating, pyrosis, sour eructations, regurgitation of food and vomiting, followed immediately by great desire for food; constipation, with headache, fullness of head, prolapsus recti after every effort of defaecation; morning diarrhoea, and then no more stool during the day; after the stools extreme weakness; colic before the stools; abdominal pains, relieved by pressure; physical and moral depression.

Continued...

Psorinum	Flat, sticky taste, the whole dinner tastes oily, tough mucus in mouth of a foul nauseous taste, the teeth stick together as if glued; dry; perfect disgust for pork; rancid eructations or tasting like rotten eggs; constant nausea during day, with inclination to vomit; vomiting of sour mucus in the morning, before eating; stitching pain pit of stomach; cutting pains in intestines; when lying down waterbrash, removed by getting up; colic removed by eating; involuntary stools at night, with much flatulency; perfect aversion to an embrace.
Ptelea trif:	Indigestion and gastric debility from hepatic troubles; mental and bodily languor; gastric headache with nausea; disgust for meat; stool in small, hard balls; netterlerash; stitches in various parts < moving, speaking, breathing; longing for acids; hepatic and gastric symptoms < after meals, feels the effect of food at once; rectal torpor.
Pulsitilla	Slow digestion, FOOD VOMITED MAY BE THAT EATEN EVEN SEVERAL DAYS BEFORE, taste of food remaining in the mouth long after eating; food tastes as if too salty, pasty or of spoiled meat, with accumulation of thick mucus in mouth; bitter taste while eating or drinking or only after swallowing food or drink; bitter a sour eructations, with sour, salty or bilious vomiting, sensation like a stone in stomach, with difficulty of breathing, especially after a meal or early on awaking; no thirst, < from cold water, heartburn, more rarely weaterbrash; frequent hiccough; feeling of tightgness after a meal, and flatulence, > by lossening clothing; bread disagrees; diarrhoea or loose stool with colicky rumbling pains in abdomen; < after ice-cream, pastry, doughnuts or anything that is fat or greasy; erratic pains in chest with gastric symptoms

Ratanhia	ATONIC DYSPEPSIA; accumulation of tasteless water in mouth; flat taste, to appetite, but constant desire to eat; eructations after dinner, empty or tasting after the ingesta; vomiting of water, preceded by loathing, empty or tasting afer the ingesta; vokiting of water, preceded by loathing; bloatedness of stomach, relieved by the emission of flatulence; coinstrictive pain in stomach, and cutting in abdomen, going off by eructations; ineffectual urging to stools, hard stools with straining; yellow diarrhoeic stools, with burning before and during stool; languor and prostration, with weariness of the whole body.
Rhus tox	(Compare with China) ATONIC DYSPEPSIA, with pain along the greater curvature of the stomach and sensation of weakness, > by exercise, somnolence, lassitude and nausea after a meal; bloatedness of the stomach, empty eructatipns; no appetite, as if one had eaten enough, with aversion to bread and meat, or desire for dainties; liquids, bread and beer disagree; frequent violent and painful eructatioins, tongue dry and thirst at night; great agitation, all his troubles area worse at night, stools preceded by colic and nearly always diarrhoeic, resesmbling jelly, or stools preceded by colic and nearly always diarrhoeic, or containing mucus and blood; hypochondriasis, meloancholy, despondency, dread of the future, > pains – by movement, rubbing, and hot applications
Ruta	After raising heavy weights eructatins after every meal accompanied by headache; pruritis of whole body; PRURITUS OF STOMACH AND INTESTINES, showing itself by pricking, gnawing pains, unquenchable desire for cold water, he rinks much and often without being incommoded by it; appetite normal, but as soon as he begins to eat aversion to everything; sudden nausea while eating, with vomiting of ingesta; difficult expulsion of the large-sized faeces, as if from want of peristaltic motion in rectum, falling of rectum.

Continued...

Rumex	Dryness of mouth and tongue during night; sensation of excoriation and of burning of the brown tongue; large quantities of dried-up mucus in pharynx, bitter taste in the morning; heaviness in the stomach, soon after eating; tasteless eructations, nausea; lanciating pains in the stomach, radiating to different points, especially forweard and to left chest; morning diarrhoea
Sabadilla	No relish for food till the first mouthful is taken, when he makes a good meal, heartburn, commencing in abdomen and extending clear up to mouth; horrid burning in stomach; empty eructations, with feeling of shuddering over body; qualmish, uncomfortable COLD sensation in stomach, nausea and desire to vomit; vomniting of ascarides, thirslessness.
Sanguinaria	RECURRING SICK-HEADACHES; flusing at the climaxis;` foetid breath, clammy sticky (Psor.) burning in throat, especially after sweet things; wants piquant articles, feels empty soon after eating, with waterbrash, lassitude almost to fainting, intense nausea after eating, in paroxysm, craves food to quiet the nausea; vomiting of sour, acrid fluids, of ingesta, of worms, soreness and pressure in epigastrium, aggravated by eating, goneness in stomach, gastro-asthenia with loss of appetite, heartburn and periodic vomiting; spasmodic constriction of cardia with gastric flatulence, exciting a feeling of tickling at the entrance of the trachea and a sympathetic dry cough; alternately constipation or diarrhoea.
Sanicula	Digestion low, can taste the food hours after eating; eructations sour, rancid, burning, fullness and bloating of stomach soon after eating, > by opening clothing and belching; nausea after eating, > after vomiting, constipation or diarrhoea. No two stools alike

Salycylic acid	FLATULENT DYSPEPSIA: extreme ditension of stomach after eating with belching up of putrid flatus, accompanied by collapse of stomach and temporary relief; vomiting characterized by the same PUTRID FERMENTATION; acidity of stomach; great irritability with despondency; anaemia.
Sarasaparilla	Loathing at the food taken; eating ever so little distends the stomach as if he had partaken of a large meal (Lyc.); feeling of emptiness, as if he had not eaten at all; much nausea; cutting and colicky pains; rumbling with sense of emptiness in abdomen; burning or cold feeling in abdomen; external abdomen very sensitive to touch; stools with much wind. Colic and backache, also after any food, as bread, which disagrees; urine dribbles away when sitting, but passes freely when standing; sand in urine or on diaper (Lyc).
Selenium	Aversion to salted food; hungry during night; great longing for ardent spirits; violent beating of pulses all over body, worse in abdomen after eating, must lie down; hard, impacted stool, needing mechanical aid for its removal; irresistible desire to lie down and sleep.
Sepia	ATONIC DYSPEPSIA, especially in women of dark complexion, suffering from portal stagnation, or incident to uterine diseases, headache, face ache, pain in stomach and abdomen after simple food; sweat of axillae or of feet exhales a very strong odour; face full of pimples; painful sensation of emptiness in stomach, with nausea as soon as she thinks of any food, heartburn extending from stomach to throat, hawking up of mucus; tongue moist and slightly fissured; taste sour, putrid, disgust for food; aversion to meat and bacon, the latter causes diarrhoea, desire for wine, beer, vinegar; nausea and great sensitiveness to any odour from cooking (cocc., colch.); sensation of a ball in stomach; sensation as if the ribs were broken and the sharp points were sticking in the flesh;

Continued...

	pressure in stomach as of a stone,< after eating, at night, pain in stomach after the simplest kind of food, acrid, sour, salty eructations, sometimes with vomiting, rumbling in abdomen after eating; sense of weight in anus, not relieved by evacuation; stools insufficient, retarded, like sheep's dung, urging to urinate from pressure on bladder, urine turbid and offensive, aversion to house-hold duties, to society; < forenoon and evening; heartbeats irregular after meal, leucorrhoea.
Silicea	Canine hunger, with nervous, irritable persons; averse to warm, cooked food, desires only cold things, disgust for meat; small quantitites of wine cause ebullitions and thirst; loud, uncontrollable, sour eructations, nausea, with violent palpitations of heart; intense heartburn, sensation of a load in epigastrium, burning or throbbing in pit stomach; morning nausea and vomiting of viscous matter; after eating, bitter taste, pressure in stomach as from a stone; flow of water in mouth; constipation, hard stools, difficult to discharge and crumbling during deffaecation.
Sinapis alba	Even the mildest food causes burning and smarting; intense burning in mouth, extending into esophagus and stomach; pit of stomach painful; ulcers on tongue, burning in esophagus with accumulations of water in mouth, causing much spitting, < afer a meal; violent heart-burn; acute bruised pain, even on light pressure, in pit of stomach, just below ensiform cartilage.
Spongia	Patient craves dainties, but after eating has dyspeptic distress and fulnes in stomach; cannot endure tight clothing around body; better from warm drinks, particularly the colicky pains in abdomen.
Staphisgria	Sensation as if STOMACH WERE HANGING DOWN RELAXED; hunger shortly after a full and substantial meal; appetite for bread and milk, for soup, wine, brandy, tobacco, feeling in abdomen as if it would drop, wants to hold it up; hot flatus, smelling like rotten eggs; stool retarded, but soft, with escape of flatus; nervous weakness: ARTHRITIS.

Stannum	Everything taste bitter or offensive but water; irregular appetite, cannot eat enough; nausea after eating, followed by vomiting of bile or undigested food; cardialgia, pains gradually come and go, extend to navel; and are better from hard pressure and walking about; sinking, gone feeling in epigastrium; rectum, much urging even with soft stool; HELMINTHIASIS; smell of cooking causes vomiting.
DYSPEPSIA REMEDIES	
Sulphur	Sinking, empty, exhausted feeling at all times without the slightest desire for food; hot flushes to face and head, frequent fainting spells; heat on vertex, with a weight as of a ton on forehead and occiput; feet icy cold. Feeling of repletion after partaking of but a small quantitiy of food; disagreeable taste when first waking up in the morning; pain of pressure and heaviness in stomach after eating; suffocation, eructations, nausea, vomiting of food early in the morning – the DYSPEPSIA OF DRUNKARDS; REGURGITATION OF FOOD; swelling of epigatrium and abdomen, pyrosis; abundant secretion of limited saliva; patient cannot digest farinaceous food, vomits milk at once; unusual hunger, with sunken and exhausted feeling at epigastrium, about 11 A.M.; very painful wind colic; constant borygmi, foetid flatus; liver engorged; constipation with frequent ineffectual desire for stool, or constipation alternating with diarrhoea; haemorrhoids; psoric diathesis; gastric ailments from REPERCUSSION OF ACUTE (ERSIPELAS) OR CHRONIC ERUPTIONS.
Sulphuric Acid	Stomach rejects water, unless it is mixed with brandy; craving for alcoholic stimulants; VOMITING OF DRUNKARDS,OF CACHECTIC PERSONS, GOING INTO STEADY DECLINE; stomach feels relaxed and cold; excessive secretion of gastric mucosities rising up into the mouth, rendering teeth dull by their acidity; sour vomit, first water, then food; debilitating diarrhoea, yellow stringy stools, having a chopped appearance.

Continued...

Tabacum	CARDIAC DYSPEPSIA; ABUSE OF TOBACCO causes dry skin; capricious appetite or none; constant desire for liquors; dull gray complextion, emaciation, hectic fever, nausea and vomiting on least motion; sticking in pit of stomach through to back; deathly nausea, with pallor, coldness; body cold, abdomen hot, paroxysms of suffocation, palpitations, intermittent beats of the heart; vertigo; irritability; great timidity; paralysis of rectum and bladder; extreme weaknes of collapse.
Taraxacum	Immoderate desire to sleep after eating; at night frightful or erotic dreams; bitter eructations for several days, returning after drinking; motions in abdomen as if bubbles were forming and bursting, hysterical tympany; debility and profuse sweat at night.
Thuja	Food testes as if it were not salt enough (Ars. Calc., cocc.): bread tastes dry and bitter (Fer., Rhus): when eating (Nitr. ac.) fatty vomiting; the fluid he drink falls audibly into the stomach (Laur.): pit of stomach sensitive to pressure, a drawing inward of the epigastrium; soreness of the umbilicus; flatulence as if an animal were crying in abdomen; motion in abdomen as if it contained something alive.
Uranium Nitricum	Vomiting of white fluid or of blood; great thirst, no appetite; tastless or putrid eructations, paroxysmal attacks of gnawing twisting pains, with sinking sensation in stomach, especially at cardia, without hunger, but relieved by food.
Veratrum Alb.	Craves fruit, juicy food, or salt food; great thirst, no appetite; tasteless or putrid eructations; heaviness after hot drinks; nausea, with sensation of fainting; violent vomiting; gastric catarrah; intestinal catarrh: especially in summer at night, with vomiting and purging, vomiting of froth, followed by vomiting of a yellow-green, sour-smelling mucus.

DYSPEPSIA REMEDIES	
Vipera torva	Nausea, vomiting, with vertigo and dyspnoea, syncope, icterus, colliquative diarrhoea, palpitations; numbness and general lassitude; dyspepsia of old people, or of persons prematurely senile, suffering from spasmodic affections of throat and chest; periodical attacks of dyspepsia
Zingiber	Vomiting of old drunkards, slimy, foul taste mornings as from disordered stomach, which feels heavy like a stone; slimy vomiting, belching and diarrhoea, cramps in soles; hot and painful haemorrhoids.
Zincum	Sweetish, metallic taste, dryness of throat; aching in pit of stomach, not much increased by pressure, terrible heartburn after taking sweets; much nawsea, vomiting and fidgety feet; as soon as the firt spoonful of food reaches the stomach it is ejected; great greediness when eating; cannot eat fast enough from canine hunger, sensation as if food lodged in esophagus, eructations with pressure at the middle of the spine; subdued nausea with tremulous feeling; < from melons, from acids or wine.
Also Refer the following remedies	
Cactus Grand	CARIAC DYSPEPSIA; indigestion; constrictive feeling at scrobiculs cordis extending to hypochondria, impending breathing; palpitate ions, felt even in temples, < ascending and walking; rumbling in stomach preceds palpitations
Cadmium sulph	Extreme tenderness of pit of stomach; spots of burning soreness in stomach and abdomen; saltish, rancid belching, cold sweat on face; cutting in stomach; nausea and vomiting of yellowish or black matter.

Continued...

Calc.carb	Chronic dyspepsia, with sensation of pressure and contraction, worse during night and after sleeping; strumous dyspepsia, with it s difficulty of assimilating fats (Eryngium): DISGUST AND REPUGNANCE FOR MEAT AND TO WARM OR COOKED FOOD, DESIRE FOR COLD VICTUALS; no appetite, continual thirst, thirst at night for cold water, but it disagrees; taste acid, bitter or putrid; tongue covered with a thick whitish-yellow coating; salivation, which eases stomach; after meal general heat, palpitation of heart, fullness and bloatedness of stomach which is sensitive to touch; eructations, without amelioration, oppression, debility and somnolence; obstinate constipation, or scanty, hard, dry stool in lumps every three or four days, or diarrhoea in scrofulous persons; urine muddy and smarting when passing; hemicrania in the morning when waking up; damp cold feet; sweats easily an nearly always cold; ill-humor and danger
Causticum	Dyspepsia of arthritic, rheumatic, haemorrhoidal patients; phlegm in throat, but inability to hawk it up; sensation of lime being burned in stomach, with rising of air; dryness of mouth, with desire to be constantly swallowing; gums sensitive and easily bleeding; paroxysmal violent pains in pit of stomach, extending into the lower abdomen and radiating into the chest back bones of the pelvis; food immediately causes heaviness and cramps; abdomen soft, only bloated by gas; constipation; vertigo when going to stool, which is hard, brown, scanty or glairy; white diarrhoea at night, with tenesmus; swollen painful haemorrhois, with pruritis ani, relieved by cold water and pressure; worse from eating fresh meat, smoked meat agrees; bread causes pressure in stomach, fat food causes offensive belching, acids cause inconvenience; water vomiting;> when stomach is empty and by lying down.

Also Refer the following remedies	
Chemomilla	Great thirst, with dry tongue; bitterness of mouth, with rising of bile and acrid eructations aggravating all pains; fullness after a meal, and afterwards nausea, vomiting of bitter green mases; heat and pain in head, red face; sensation of burning in eyes, agitated sleep, with great irritation, bloated abdomen, colic, with green diarrhoeic stools, embarrassed respiration.
Dioscorea	Pain and spasm arise from the umbilical region and radiate all over abdomen, extending into stomach, pelvic organs and even extremities; sharp cramping pains in pit of stomach, followed by raising, belching and gulping enormous quantities of tasteless wind, followed by hiccough and discharge of flatus downward, with sensation as if both temples were in vise; must unfasten clothing; dull, heavy, weary pain in stomach, with faintness; haemorrhoids.
Moschus	Persistent troubles of digestive functions in susceptible hysterical persons, with palpitation of heart, dyspnoea and prostration; is afraid to lie down for fear of death.
Mur. Acid	HABITUAL DIFFICULT DIGESTION; EVERYTHING TASTES SWEET; acrid and putrid taste, like rotten eggs, with ptyalism; excessive hunger and thirst, morbid longing for alcoholic drinks, aversion to meat; bitter, putrid eructations; vomiting, with belching, coughing; involuntary swallowing, gulping of contents of stomach into esophagus, which sometimes go down again; empty sensation in stomach, extending through the whole abdomen; weak feeling in stomach, but no hunger; stool difficult, as from inactivity of bowels; prostration and drowsiness all day, wants to lie about peevishness
Nat. Carb	HYPOCHONDRIASIS DURING DIGESTION; dyspepsia > by eating soda biscuits; tongue red, mucous surface smooth and shining; burning pain and tensioin from pit of stomach often with colicky pain soon after eating, with mucous relaxation of the bowels; sour eructations, waterbrash, retching in the morning with spasmodic contraction of both esophagus and stomach,

Continued...

	with nothing coming up, but copious salivation; stitches in liver and spleen, abundant expulsion of foetid flatus; constipation alternating with soft or liquid stools, vegetables and starchy food is badly digested (Magn. Carb), weariness of life.
Plumbum	Lead dyspepsia in persons suffering already with numbness of the extremities; intolerable pain in stomach, pressing, burning, stitching, tearing, sour, greenish, blackish vomiting; copious vomitting of thick, white fluid, which falls in a trembling mass, like the white of an egg; hot and foetid eructatioins; tongue yellow, coated, or dry, brown and fissured; lips excoriated; total loss of appetite alternating with bulimy, even after taking a meal; beating and burning; pains of constriction in stomach, which meet around the navel; abdominal walls hard, contracted; umblicus sunken in; stubborn constipation; with constant desire to go to stool without any result; stools voluminous hard, expelled only with great force, commonly environed with mucus, or sanguinolent, yellow dioarrhoea, of very bad odor; emaciatioin.
Robinia	Food, soon after eating, turns sour; constant feeling of weight in stomach, with fulnes and tension; eructations, accompanied by a sour liquid, with vomiting, at times, of portions of the ingesta; burning pain in stomach and between scapulae; thirst; constant frontal headache; water taken worse at night preventing sleep, EXCESSIVE ACIDITY OF STOMACH, vomiting of intensely sour fluid, setting the teeth on edge; great distension of stomach and bowels with flatulence; sour vomiting of infants, the whole child smells sour (Rheum); desire for stool, but only flatulence passes off; constipation; constant dull headache, < buy motion; low spirtits.

NERVOUS DYSPEPSIA

Synonyms: Atonic dyspepsia, gastric neurasthenia

Aetiology: The neurosis occurs most commonly in those between the ages of twenty and forty, but may occur earlier or later in life. The exciting cases are overwork, excitement, care worry, sorrow, sexual excesses, and improper manner of living. In some cases the patient to be robust, but on more careful examination is found to present nervous symptoms.

Symptoms: These are indefinite, capricious and changeable. There is hyperasthesea or a diffused sensitiveness confined to the area of the stomach. The changeable appetite alternates with constipation and diarrhea, and a feeling of general depression, sleeplessness and ill humor and fatigue are present. During the morning there is a sensation of illness and pressure about the head, vomiting is often present and is dependent upon a spasm of the pylorus.

NERVOUS DYSPEPSIA: (Remedies)	
Anacardim	Indicated when there is great accumulation of gas with frequent eructations and a sensation of wean sand sinking in the epigstrium extending to the spine. This distress, similar to that of *Kali phos*, occurs as soon as the stomach is empty, or partially empty, and is relieved by eating. The patient complains of hearing voices, and being conscious of a double ego, and desire to curse and swear
Cuprum Ars	Is frequently of service when there is a history of improper diet. The patient complains of distress and cramping pains that extend to the extremities, and is weak, anemic and debilitated.
China Off	Sexual excesses –especially after effects of loss of semen due to masturbation as these effects continue almost life long – Flatulence, distension of stomach and abdomen especially after eating – like load tight feeling – must loosen the clothes to get relief – Humming/Roaming in the ears –– even soft stool is passed with difficulty – pain> by hard pressure (*To be taken half an hour before food*)

Continued...

Kali phos	Should be studied in neurasthenic subjects who complain of an all-gone sensation of the stomach temporarily relieved by eating. The gastric symptoms are aggravated by excitement and worry. The urine is diminished in quantity and contains an excess of phosphates. It is frequently found curative when Anacardium has failed to relieve.
Nat Mur	Nervous dyspepsia in the persons who are habituated to masturbation and adverse effects of masturbation.
Strychnine Phos – 6	Is better who are engaged with mental strain, have their meals at irregular hours, who do not masticate their food thoroughly and are not careful of the quality of the food. They are irritable, depressed and suffer from insomnia and palpitation of the heart. There is a bad taste in the mouth, the tongue is coated and there is frontal headache. The patient craves cold and acid drinks and following the meals there is nausea and vomiting of sour fluid and partially digested foods.

ACUTE CATARRHAL GASTRITIS

Symptoms: The disease shows all grades of severity, appetite is lost, there is a sour, disagreeable taste in the mouth and the patient shows aversion to food. Tongue is covered with thick greyish coating, somewhat swollen, and the margins show indentation of the teeth. A sense of weight is complained in the epigastric region. There is also nausea and vomiting of sour, foul, partially digested food and more or less mucus with vomited material, which is acid in reaction and may appear swollen. Patient complains of lassitude, headache, usually with vertigo. Urine is highly coloured, decreased in amount, contains uric acid and often indican. As a rule, no fever, but the pulse is rapid small and compressible.

Mild cases recover within a few days. In the more severe forms the vomiting continues while disturbance may extend to the bowels, and as a result constipation which is usually present gives place to diarrhoea.

When the duodenum becomes affected, jaundice may occur. If fever should be present, it is usually remittent in character, and herpes labialis may appear.

ACUTE CATARRHAL GASTRITIS: (Remedies)	
Ars. Alb.	Indicated in acute gastric catarrh, when there is violent vomiting of everything ingested. There are severe burning pains referred to the stomach. The stomach is sensitive and sore and the patient is greatly prostrated. The gastritis may terminate in ulceration
Ant. Crud.	Indicate when the attack has been produced by overeating. The stomach is weak and digestion is easily disturbed. There is a thick, milk-white coating on the tongue. The trouble is aggravated by bread, pastry, acids, especially vinegar, sour or bad wine, from hot weather, overeating and often cold bathing.
Bry. Alb.	Useful in hot weather, when an attack is the result of taking cold drinks when heated. There are sticking pains in stomach which are worse from motion. Tongue is coated white or a dark brownish yellow. Lips are dry and there is either lack of thirst or an intense and constant thirst for large quantities of water. Stools are large and dry and have the appearance of being burnt.
Graphites	Has a favourable action on many of these cases when there is vomiting of food with bitter, sour regurgitation of food. The stomach is dilated in many of these cases. The patient is inclined to obesity and suffers from habitual constipation. If the patient is woman, there is a history of delayed menstruation. In many cases the skin presents an unhealthy cracked appearance.
Hydrastis	Indicated in acute attacks, especially of beer drinkers, when there is loss of appetite with sour eructation. There is yellow coating in the centre of the tongue, while the tip and sides are clean. The patient complains of lassitude, malaise and depression of spirits. The liver is enlarged and sensitive, and there is slight jaundice. The bowels are usually constipated.

Continued...

Ipecauc.	Indicated when there is a constant nausea easy vomiting, constant eructation and accumulations of saliva in the mouth. The vomiting gives no relief. The tongue is clear or slightly coated. There is a sensation as though the stomach were relaxed and hanging, and clutching, squeezing, griping pains as if each finger of a hand were pressing sharply into the intestines. These symptoms are worse from motion.
Nux. Vom.	When there have been errors of diet, with irregular habits, close confinement, mental over exertion, loss of sleep and debauchery. The bowels are constipated and there are ineffectual efforts to stool, with hemorrhoids. The tongue is coated white, and there is a dull frontal headache. The complexion is sallow and there are bitter, sour eructation, hiccough and heartburn. There is vomiting of food, mucus and bile. The patient is always worse an hour or two after eating a hearty meal and is irritable and cross.
Phosphorous	Vomits as soon as food enters the stomach. He craves cold food and cold drinks which relieve momentarily, but are vomited as soon as they become warm in the stomach. There is often a weak, all gone sensation in the stomach at 11 a.m which extends the bowels.
Pulsatilla	In cases that are brought on by the use of ice cream, fruits or rich pastry. The tongue is white or yellow and there is no appetite and no thirst, even if the mouth is dry and parched. There is a bitter taste in the month and the sides of the tongue feel scalded. The patient has an aversion to fats, milk, butter, meat, and hot foods and by confinement in closed warm rooms.

CHRONIC GASTRITIS

Synonyms: Chronic gastric catarrh, Chronic Dyspepsia.

Symptoms:

This is a chronic condition of the mucous membrane of the stomach, which may extend to the deep coats, and is associated with an increased quantity of mucus, qualitative and quantitative changes, in the gastric juice, and deficient motility of the stomach. There is frequently a sensation of gastric fullness after eating which may be accompanied by nausea and vomiting, eructation of sour gases, and palpitation. The tongue is moist and has greyish white fur, while its tip and margin are red. Pressure over the epigastric region elicits pain. Pain is also complained of after swallowing food. There is a gradual loss of weight and secondary anemia with the advancement of the disease. The appetite is variable and at times there is a craving for certain kinds of food. There are burning eructations of gas and of bitter sour fluid. The bowels are obstinately constipated. Headache, mental depression melancholia and irritability are present and cough often accompanies the disease. The amount of hydrochloric acid secreted is reduced and may be absent, interfering with the digestion of proteids. Pepsin and the curdling ferment, while rarely absent, may be greatly reduced. There is a large amount of mucus in the stomach.

The motor power of the stomach is decreased as the disease progresses so that the food is retained hours longer than it should be, resulting in a hyperacidity of the contents, together with fermentation and decomposition. Dilation of the stomach gradually follows and in turn increases the motor insufficiency of the stomach. The disturbance of the nervous mechanism of the stomach is manifested in a variety of ways, as irritability of the mucosa. In other cases there is a sensation of weight or pain, or capricious appetite. s The general metabolism is interfered with and emaciation results.

Examination of the gastric contents following administration of a test meal, shows large quantities of mucus, hydrochloric acid is diminished, or may be absent, though occasionally it is present in normal quantities. If there is a large quantity of mucus, lactic acid is usually present.

CHRONIC GASTRITIS – Remedies	
Ars. Alb.	Restlessness, anxiety, thirst, and a sensation of burning in the epigastric region. In many of these cases in which this remedy indicated with a history of alcoholism that has produced gastric irritability and vomiting. In connection with this remedy **Chin. Ars. and Ars.iod. should be studied.**
Arg. Nitricum	Excessive flatulence. There is belching after each meal, with distension of the stomach as though it would burst. The belching is difficult, finally the air rushes out with great violence. There is vomiting of a large quantity of ropy mucus.
Acid Carbolic	Excessive flatulence, acid eructation, nausea and vomiting shortly after eating. If vomiting does not take place there are pains in the stomach and abdomen during digestion. The tongue is red, thick and slightly coated at the base. The patient complains off a sensation of goneness after meals.
Bismuth subnitrate	Cases characterized by a sweetish metallic taste in the mouth. There is a thirst for cold drinks but the cold water taken is immediately vomited and a sensation of burning in the stomach after meals. This is confined to a small circumscribed spot. The patient desires to bend backward. Nausea, flatulence and eructation of an offensive odour. The bowels may be constipated or there may be an alternate constipation and diarrhoea.
Bry. Alb.	To be studied when there is an offensive, flat, bitter taste in the mouth and white coated tongue. Sensation as of a stone in the stomach and is aggravated by motion. The digestive process is slow. Bowels are constipated, e stools are dry and dark brown as if burnt. The liver is sensitive to palpitation.

Bismuth subgallate	Cases characterized by fermentation, slow digestion and an excess of gas and flatulence
Bry. Alb.	To be studied when there is an offensive, flat, bitter taste in the mouth and white coated tongue. Sensation as of a stone in the stomach and is aggravated by motion. The digestive process is slow. Bowels are constipated, e stools are dry and dark brown as if burnt. The liver is sensitive to palpitation.
Carbo veg	In weak, debilitated patients who complain of great flatulence. The simplest food disagrees, everything seems to turn to gas. The abdomen is distended and there is a rumbling of gas and the passage of much flatus with foul odour. Soreness and cramping pain in the epigastrium, oppressed breathing and palpitation of the heart in consequence of the fullness and oppression.
Hydrastis	Acute attacks, especially of beer drinkers, when there is loss of appetite with sour eructation. There is a yellow coating in the centre of the tongue, while the tip and sides are clean. The patient complaints of lassitude, malaise and depression of spirits. The liver is enlarged and sensitive and there is slight jaundice. The bowels are usually constipated.
Ipecacac	Indicated when there is constant nausea easy vomiting, eructation and accumulations of saliva in the mouth. Vomiting gives no relief. The tongue is clear or slightly coated. Sensation as though the stomach were relaxed and hanging down, clutching, squeezing, griping pains as if each finger of a hand were pressing sharply into the intestines. These symptoms are worse from motion.
Kreosutum	Food is retained in the stomach and is then vomited unchanged, showing that digestion has practically ceased. It is especially useful when tuberculosis is present.

Continued...

Lycopodium	Subjects, where Uric Acid levels are high, complain of sudden repletion when eating so that they are unable to eat enough to satisfy their hunger nor as much as the system needs. There is great fermentation in the abdomen with rumbling and cracking noises. There is colic and discharge of much flatus which worse from 4 to 8 p.m
Nux Vom	This is indicated in which medicines, purgatives and laxatives have been taken previously by the patients. The patient is drowsy during the evening, is restless during the last part of the night, and is worse in the morning. Tongue is furred, the breath is foul and retches and vomits. The bowels are constipated and there is ineffectual urging to stool. The patient is irritable and peevish. In some cases it will be found that Strychnine acts better, especially if motor insufficiency is prominent symptom
Pusatilla	Patients with a changeable, peevish disposition. They are easily moved to tears and laughter, and are of a silent temperament, disgusted at everything. Complain of a headache from overloading the stomach with pastry, fats or ice cream. The digestion is slow, foods ferment and as a result there are eructation and flatulence.
Sepia	Indicated in neurotic women who suffer from uterine diseases. She complains of acid eructation, changeable appetite and a desire for such articles of diet as will act as stimulants. She complains of sensation of burning in the epigastric region following meals which may simulate gastralgia. The urine has a putrid odour and contains a large amount of urates.

Flatulency (Gas in Intestines of stomach – Remedies	
Carbo-veg	When the gas is coming upwards wit relief by belching – burning pains
China	Incarcerated flatus – there is stagnation of gas without relief by belching – Loss of animal fluids i.e. blood, semen and water etc.
Lycopodium	When gas is more in intestines and coming downwards
Raphanus	Gas either comes up or goes down

GASTRALGIA

Synonyms: – Gastrodynia, Cardialgia, Neuralgia of the stomach

Definition & Etiology:

An affection of the sensory filaments of the pneumogastric nerve characterised by severe boring painful contraction in the epigastric region, that extends from the xiphoid cartilage and radiates to the back. It may be accompanied by syncope and signs of collapse. This affection is associated most frequently with a central neurosis as hysteria and neurasthenia, or a motor or secondary neurosis, pylorospasm, cardiospasm, gastro-succorrhea, or it may have a central cause in tabes dorsalis. In some cases it is the result of reflex influences as displaced uterus, an inflamed ovary, or an ovarian neoplasm. Mental over-exertion, wasting, discharges, excessive indulgence in alcohol, tea, coffee, tobacco and sexual excesses for its development. Peritoneal adhesions between the stomach, pancreas, liver or spleen have also been known to be the exciting cause.

Symptoms:

This affection is characterized by intense, agonizing pain in the epigastrium. This may appear while the stomach is empty, again shortly after a meal, and especially if articles of diet or drink have been taken that are not well borne, even in a condition of health. It may be precipitated by a psychic condition, or it may occur in women during the menstrual period. The pain appears more or less suddenly and may be a so severe as to cause a reflex spasm of the cutaneous vessels. The skin becomes pale, is covered with cold, clammy sweat, and syncope and clonic muscular contractions may occur. The pulse is small, the patient moans, bends forward and presses upon the abdomen. There may be but one attack, but more frequently they are recurrent and may persist for months.

GASTRALGIA (remedies)	
Acid oxalic	Neurasthenic subjects. The pains have periods of remission, worse from motion and while thinking about them. Gastralgia appears after eating, with pyrosis and cold feeling externally between epigastrium and umbilicus.
Ars. Alb	Those who complain extreme weakness and prostration, or acute burning, or gnawing, corroding pains accompanied by great restlessness, nervous excitability, coldness of the extremities, palpitation of the heart and aggravations; feeling as if the stomach were inflamed; pressure in the stomach with pale face and earthy complexion; induced by eating ice cream, cake etc.
Bryonia alb	Rheumatic diathesis who are of bilious tendency, irritable and incline to anger, complain contractive, pinching pains, relieved by eructations; pressure in the stomach after eating as from a stone; soreness and tenderness in the epigastrium; bloated feeling in the stomach, with stitches and oppression of breathing; symptoms aggravated by motion and by eating; pains on in chronic cases an hour or two after eating and continue for several hours.

Belladona	Gastralgia that appears suddenly. There are cramping or shooting pains in the pit of the stomach, forcing the patient to bend backward and to hold his breath; periodical pains in the pit of the stomach, with tremor; region of the stomach sensitive to the touch face bloated and congested; pressing, drawing and clutching pains extending to the back, nausea, thirst and vomiting, aggravated by drinking water or by motion, and ameliorated by eating.
Bismuth Subnitricum	Cases of gastralgia when there is burning, griping, lancinating pain in the epigastrium with pressure in the stomach as from a load; burning pain in the stomach extending to the spine, with waterbrash, flatulence and extreme pain in the stomach, extending to the spine, pains are sometimes relieved by bending backward.
Carbo veg	Fermentive dyspepsia with acidity and gastralgia, waterbrash, coming on about 3 p.m. with thirst for cold water, bloating of the stomach, with burning pains, relieved by eructation; vomiting of large quantities of mucus tinged with bile, giving relief; suited to cases complicated with hysteria or dyspepsia, especially if there is present, a hyperaemic and irritable condition of the lining membrane of the stomach.
Colocynthis	Paroxsimal pains that extend into the umbilical region, obliging the patient to bend double; exacerbations recur every few minutes, are not the result of indigestion but rather, in some cases, of emotional excitement.
Cocculus Indicus	Indicated in those who suffer from spasmodic and flatulent colic with cramping pains in the stomach, preventing sleep, violent pinching, griping and cramping pains in the epigastric region, great distension of the stomach from accumulation of gases; especially suited to cases where Nux Vom., being indicated, fails to cure, pyrosis is not present.

Continued...

China	Indicated in those who have become debilitated as a result of exhausting discharges, loss of vital fluids. The gastralgia is attended with great chilliness or coldness; constant feeling of weariness and debility, heartburn, with sour eructations bloated abdomen and palpitation of the heart; gastralgia at a certain hour every day or every other day; gastralgia after natural or artificial depletions; torpid liver, with jaundiced hue, and large, undigested stools, worse at night; pains aggravated or excited by cold, eating, or by emotions.
Fer met.	In those who are anaemic and suffer from atony of the stomach; heartburn, with feeling of a load in the stomach; vomiting immediately after eating, which usually relieves the suffering; aggravated or induced by coughing and moving about.
Ignatia	Nervous hysterical patients, especially females who are introspective, silent, melancholy given to sighing and weeping. There are cramping pains in the stomach, sharp, pinching, pressing pains in the pit of the stomach and in the right hypochondrium; pressive pain in the epigastrium; a relaxed flabby feeling in the stomach, or an all-gone feeling, as if from fasting, with great exhaustion; hysterical, changeful moods, now tearful, silent and melancholy, then impatient, irresolute, ill – humoured and angry; burning in the stomach, regurgitation of food, frequent voiding of large quantities of pale urine.
Nux.vom	In cases characterized by cramping, spasmodic pain. The patient is of irritable, careful, jealous type, with dark hair; bilious of sanguine temperament and is disposed to be quarrelsome, spiteful, malicious, nervous and melancholy, and especially sensitive to pain. In the majority of these cases the patient has been taking an excessive amount of tea, coffee tobacco, or alcoholic stimulants

Ran. Bulb	Gastralgia pain as from excoriation and burning sensation in pit of stomach as also in cardiac end (orifice) of stomach especially when parts are touched (inflammation of stomach) erosion? – Immediately after eating violent stitches from left lumbar region transversely through abdomen, especially below umbilicus and towards right.
Pulsatilla	In those who are slow and indecisive. Their symptoms are always changing. They complain of heartburn when the stomach is empty; sour and bitter vomiting, with absence of thirst, feeling as if food had lodged in the eseophagus; indigestion proved or aggravated by eating of rich of fat food.
Vertrum Alb	Indicated in those who are always chilly and complain of a cold perspiration, especially upon the forehead. There is pain in the epigastrium, coming on gradually, radiating upward to both sides and to the back between the scapulae, increasing in violence till it becomes agonizing, then gradually wearing off; especially adapted to those cases in which the celiac plexus and sympathetic are involved; pain increases and subsides gradually, and is attended with marked coldness of the extremities.

GASTRIC HYPERESTHSIA

Definition:

This is a gastric neurosis characterized by increased irritability of the sensory nerves of the stomach which gives rise to a sensation of fullness, tension and oppression in the gastric region, after food. In some cases the distress is so intense that the patient refuses any food.

Aetiology:

This is dependent upon a neurosis in hypochondrical subjects. It is often associated with chlorosis, while excess of alcohol or venery may be predisposing causes. It has been observed in cases of hyperacidity and locomotor ataxia.

Symptoms:

There is an increased irritability of the stomach so that the mildest food causes a painful sensation. This may be in the form of heat or cold, gnawing, pulling or burning, and the taking of least food causes distress, even nausea and vomiting, again it may be relieved by taking food.

GASTRIC HYPERESTHSIA: (Remedies)	
Ar. Nit. 6	15 minutes before food.
Ars Alb	Should be studied when the patient complains of the burning, thirst and restlessness that characterizes the remedy.
Bismuth Subnit.	Should be remembered when the pain and distress is pronounced
Chinium Ars.	Is indicated when there is a sensation of burning and soreness in the stomach

GERD, or Gastroesophageal Reflux Disease –

Occurs when the lower esophageal sphincter is not able to close properly. When this happens, contents from the stomach, called reflux, leak back into the esophagus and the stomach.

When the stomach refluxes, stomach acid touches the lining of the esophagus and causes it to have a burning feeling in the throat or the chest. This is what heartburn is. When you taste the fluid in the back of your throat, it is called acid indigestion. It is common for a person to get occasional heartburn, but when it occurs more than twice a week it can be considered to be GERD. GERD can occur in people of all ages including infants.

Some symptoms of GERD include having a pain in your chest, hoarseness, having trouble swallowing, or having the feeling of food being stuck in your throat. The main symptoms are having persistent heartburn and acid regurgitation. GERD can also cause bad breath and a dry cough.

No one knows why people get GERD. Some things that could contribute to GERD are alcohol use, pregnancy, being overweight and smoking. Certain foods might also contribute like citrus fruits, caffeine, spicy, fatty, and dried foods, and also mint flavourings. Over-the-counter antacids or medications that help stop acid production and help the muscles empty the stomach are commonly used to treat GERD.

HYPERCHLORHYDRIA

Before studying on **HYPERCHLORHYDRIA** go through the following natural ways to prevent Heart burn and Acid Reflux: The most frequently used treatment involves commercial medications, such as omeprazole. However, lifestyle modifications may be effective as well. Simply changing dietary habits or the way of sleeping may significantly reduce symptoms of heartburn and acid reflux, improving quality of life.

What Is Acid Reflux and its Symptoms? – – – When stomach acid gets pushed up into the esophagus, the tube that carries food and drink from **the mouth to the stomach**. Some reflux is totally normal and harmless, usually causing no symptoms. But when it happens too often, it burns inside of the esophagus. **It is estimated 14–20% of all** adults in US have reflux in some form or another. The most common symptom of acid reflux is known as heartburn, which is a painful, burning feeling in the chest or throat. Researchers estimate that around 7% of Americans experience heartburn daily. Of those who regularly experience heartburn, 20–40% are diagnosed with gastroesophageal reflux disease (GERD), which is the most serious form of acid reflux. GERD is the most common digestive disorder in the US.

In addition to heartburn, common symptoms of reflux include an acidic taste at the back of the mouth and difficulty swallowing. Other symptoms include a cough, asthma, tooth erosion and inflammation in the sinuses. So here are 14 natural ways to reduce your acid reflux and heartburn, all backed by scientific research.

1. Heavy eating to be avoided: Where the esophagus opens into the stomach, there is a ring-like **muscle known as the lower esophageal sphincter.** It acts as a valve and is supposed to prevent the acidic contents of the stomach from going up into the esophagus. It naturally opens when you swallow, belch or vomit. Otherwise, it should stay closed.

In people with acid reflux, this muscle is weakened or dysfunctional. Acid reflux can also occur when there is too much pressure on the muscle, causing acid to squeeze through the opening. Unsurprisingly, most reflux symptoms take place after a meal. It also seems that larger meals may worsen reflux symptoms. One step that will help minimize acid reflux is to avoid eating large meals.

SUMMARY: Avoid eating large meals. Acid reflux usually increases after meals, and larger meals seem to make the problem worse.

2. Loose Weight: The diaphragm is a muscle located above your stomach. In healthy people, the diaphragm naturally strengthens the lower esophageal sphincter. As mentioned earlier, this muscle prevents excessive amounts of stomach acid from leaking up into the esophagus. However, if you have too much *belly fat* the pressure in your abdomen may become so high that the lower esophageal sphincter gets pushed upward, away from the diaphragm's support. This condition is known as hiatus hernia. – **Hiatus hernia** is the main reason for obese people and pregnant women are at an increased risk of reflux and heartburn. Several observational studies show that extra pounds in the abdominal area increase the risk of reflux and GERD. Controlled studies support this, showing that weight loss may relieve reflux symptoms. Losing weight should be one of your priorities if you live with acid reflux.

SUMMARY: Excessive pressure inside the abdomen is one of the reasons for acid reflux. Losing belly fat might relieve some of your symptoms.

3. Follow a Low-Carb Diet (i.e. carbo hydrates):

Growing evidence suggests that *low carb diets* relieve acid reflux symptoms. Scientists suspect that undigested carbs may be causing bacterial overgrowth and elevated pressure inside the abdomen. Some even speculate this may be one of the most common causes of acid reflux. Studies indicate that bacterial overgrowth is caused by impaired carb digestion and absorption. Having too many undigested carbs in digestive system makes gassy and bloated. It also tends to belch more often. Supporting this idea, a few small studies indicate that low-carb diets improve reflux symptoms. Additionally, an antibiotic treatment may significantly reduce acid reflux, possibly by decreasing the numbers of gas-producing bacteria. In one study, researchers gave participants with GERD **prebiotic fiber** supplements that promoted the growth of gas-producing bacteria. The participants› reflux symptoms worsened as a result.

SUMMARY: Acid reflux might be caused by poor carb digestion and bacterial overgrowth in the small intestine. Low-carb diets appear to be an effective treatment, but further studies are needed.

4. Limit Alcohol Intake: Drinking alcohol may increase the severity of acid reflux and heartburn. It aggravates symptoms by increasing stomach acid, relaxing the lower esophageal sphincter and impairing the ability of the esophagus to clear itself of acid. Studies have shown that moderate alcohol intake may even cause reflux symptoms in healthy individuals. Controlled studies also show that drinking wine or beer increases reflux symptoms, compared to drinking plain water.

SUMMARY: Excessive alcohol intake can worsen acid reflux symptoms. If you experience heartburn, limiting your alcohol intake might help ease some of your pain.

5. Don't Drink Too Much Coffee: Studies show that coffee temporarily weakens the lower esophageal sphincter, increasing the risk of acid reflux. Some evidence points towards caffeine as a possible culprit. Similar to coffee, caffeine weakens the lower esophageal sphincter. Additionally, drinking decaffeinated coffee has been shown to reduce reflux compared to regular coffee.

However, one study that gave participants caffeine in water was unable to detect any effects of caffeine on reflux, even though coffee itself worsened the symptoms. These findings indicate that compounds other than caffeine may play a role in coffee's effects on acid reflux. The processing and preparation of coffee might also be involved. Nevertheless, although several studies suggest that coffee may worsen acid reflux, the evidence is not entirely conclusive.

One study found no adverse effects when acid reflux patients consumed coffee right after meals, compared to an equal amount of warm water. However, coffee increased the duration of reflux episodes between meals. Additionally, an analysis of observational studies found no significant effects of coffee intake on the self-reported symptoms of GERD. Yet, when the signs of acid reflux were investigated with a small camera, coffee consumption was linked with greater acid damage in the esophagus. Whether coffee intake worsens acid reflux may depend on the individual. If coffee gives you heartburn, simply avoid it or limit your intake.

SUMMARY: Evidence suggests that coffee makes acid reflux and heartburn worse. If you feel like coffee increases your symptoms, you should consider limiting your intake.

6. Chew Gum: A few studies show that chewing gum reduces acidity in the esophagus... Gum that contains bicarbonate appears to be especially effective. These findings indicate that chewing gum — and the associated increase in saliva production — may help clear the esophagus of acid. However, it probably doesn›t reduce the reflux itself.

SUMMARY: Chewing gum increases the formation of saliva and helps clear the esophagus of stomach acid.

7. Avoid Raw Onion: One study in people with acid reflux showed that eating a meal containing raw onion significantly increased heartburn, acid reflux and belching compared with an identical meal that didn't contain onion. More frequent belching might suggest that more gas is being produced due to the high amounts of fermentable fiber in onions. Raw onions might also irritate the lining of the esophagus, causing worsened heartburn. Whatever the reason, if you feel like eating raw onion makes your symptoms worse, you should avoid it.

SUMMARY: Some people experience worsened heartburn and other reflux symptoms after eating raw onion.

8. Limit Your Intake of Carbonated Beverages: Patients with GERD are sometimes advised to limit their intake of carbonated beverages. One observational study found that carbonated soft drinks were associated with increased acid reflux symptoms. Also, controlled studies show that drinking carbonated water or cola temporarily weakens the lower esophageal sphincter, compared to drinking plain water. The main reason is the carbon dioxide gas in carbonated beverages, which causes people to belch more often — an effect that can increase the amount of acid escaping into the esophagus.

SUMMARY: Carbonated beverages temporarily increase the frequency of belching, which may promote acid reflux. If they worsen your symptoms, try drinking less or avoiding them altogether.

9. Don't Drink Too Much Citrus Juice: In a study of 400 GERD patients, 72% reported that orange or grapefruit juice worsened their acid reflux symptoms. The acidity of citrus fruits doesn't appear to be the only factor contributing to these effects. Orange juice with a neutral pH also appears to aggravate symptoms.

Since citrus juice doesn't weaken the lower esophageal sphincter, it is likely that some of its constituents irritate the lining of the esophagus... While citrus juice probably doesn't cause acid reflux, it can make your heartburn temporarily worse.

SUMMARY: Most patients with acid reflux report that drinking citrus juice makes their symptoms worse. Researchers believe citrus juice irritates the lining of the esophagus.

10. Consider Eating Less Chocolate: GERD patients are sometimes advised to avoid or limit their consumption of chocolate. However, the evidence for this recommendation is weak. One small, uncontrolled study showed that consuming 4 ounces (120 ml) of chocolate syrup weakened the lower esophageal sphincter. Another controlled study found that drinking a chocolate beverage increased the amount of acid in the esophagus, compared to a placebo. Nevertheless, further studies are needed before any strong conclusions can be made about the effects of chocolate on reflux symptoms.

SUMMARY: There is limited evidence that chocolate worsens reflux symptoms. A few studies suggest it might, but more research is needed.

Get Answers from a Doctor in Minutes, Anytime Have medical questions? Connect with a board-certified, experienced doctor online or by phone. Pediatricians and other specialists available 24/7.

11. Avoid Mint – If Needed Refer to Doctor: Peppermint and spearmint are common herbs used to flavor foods, candy, chewing gum, mouthwash and toothpaste. They are also popular ingredients in herbal teas. One controlled study of patients with GERD found no evidence for the effects of spearmint on the lower esophageal sphincter. Yet, the study showed that high doses of spearmint may worsen acid reflux symptoms, presumably by irritating the inside of the esophagus. If you feel like mint makes your heartburn worse, then avoid it.

SUMMARY: A few studies indicate that mint may aggravate heartburn and other reflux symptoms, but the evidence is limited.

12. Elevate the Head of Your Bed: Some people experience reflux symptoms during the night. This may disrupt their sleep quality and make it difficult for them to fall asleep. One study showed that patients who raised the head of their bed had significantly fewer reflux episodes and symptoms, compared to those who slept without any elevation. Additionally, an analysis of controlled studies concluded that elevating the head of the bed is an effective strategy to reduce acid reflux symptoms and heartburn at night...

SUMMARY: Elevating the head of your bed may reduce your reflux symptoms at night.

13. Don't Eat Within Three Hours of Going to Bed: People with acid reflux are generally advised to avoid eating within the three hours before they go to sleep. Although this recommendation makes sense, there is limited evidence to back it up. One study in GERD patients showed that having a late evening meal had no effects on acid reflux, compared to having a meal before 7 p.m. (50Trusted Source).

However, an observational study found that eating close to bedtime was associated with significantly greater reflux symptoms when people were going to sleep **(51Trusted Source)**. More studies are needed before solid conclusions can be made about the effect of late evening meals on GERD. It may also depend on the individual.

SUMMARY: Observational studies suggest that eating close to bedtime may worsen acid reflux symptoms at night. Yet, the evidence is inconclusive and more studies are needed.

14. Don't Sleep on Your Right Side: Several studies show that sleeping on your right side may worsen reflux symptoms at night. The reason is not entirely clear, but is possibly explained by anatomy. The esophagus enters the right side of the stomach. As a result, the lower esophageal sphincter sits above the level of stomach acid when you sleep on your left side.

When you lay on your right side, stomach acid covers the lower esophageal sphincter. This increases the risk of acid leaking through it and causing reflux. Obviously, this recommendation may not be practical, since most people change their position while they sleep. **Yet resting on your left side might make you more comfortable as you fall asleep.**

SUMMARY: If you experience acid reflux at night, avoid sleeping on the right side of your body.

The Bottom Line:

Some scientists claim that dietary factors are a major underlying cause of acid reflux. While this might be true, more research is needed to substantiate these claims. Nevertheless, studies show that simple dietary and lifestyle changes can significantly ease heartburn and other acid reflux symptoms.

HYPERCHLORHYDRIA (Remedies)	
Arg. Nit.	Is useful in neurotic patients in whom there is great distension of the stomach, and violent eructations of gas, which comes up with force, after which the patient feels relieved. There is severe pain in many cases. The patient is exhausted, though the food is not vomited – it does not appear to nourish the patient to any extent.
Acid Sulph	Acidity of alcoholics or even in all cases hyperchlordia
Graphites	When the digestion is slow and imperfect, there are accumulations of gas in the bowel with much distension and vomiting of sour material. The tongue is coated, there is a bitter taste in the mouth, with eructations of sour fluid. The bowels are constipated, stools are large and knotty and are evacuated with difficulty, or they may consist of partially digested food and have a putrid odour.

Hydrastis	Cases which are accompanied by chronic gastritis and atonic dyspepsia, torpidity of the liver, enfeebled circulation and constipation. The appetite is poor and there is gastric distress especially after eating bread and vegetables. There are sour eructations and a sensation as of weight in the stomach or of emptiness and an all-gone sensation.
Ipecac	Cases in which there is persistent nausea and vomiting and more or less abdominal colic which is characterized by a griping pain as though the intestines were grasped by a hand.
Iris verse	Indicated in cases where there is great burning and distress in the region of the stomach. There are sour eructations nausea and vomiting of intensely sour material. The patient is subject to sick headache which begin with a blur before the eyes.
Nat Carb	Feels swollen and sensitive stomach. Ill effects of drinking cold water when overheated. Very weak digestion, caused by slightest error of diet. Depressed after eating. Bitter taste in old Dyspeptics, always belching, sour stomach and rheumatism. Dyspepsia relieved by soda biscuits.
Nux-vom.	Hypochhondridal subjects, who give a history of gastric and liver complaints, live a sedentary life, whose diet contains highly seasoned foods, and excess of coffee, tea and spirituous liquors. The tongue is red and tender, coated yellow at the base and there are excessive acid eructations or vomiting of sour fluid. Nausea and vomiting each morning. The bowels are usually constipated. The stools are large and difficult to evacuate, but with frequent urging.
Robinea	Indicated in cases characterized by excessive acidity of the stomach. Acid eructations in the early morning during empty stomach with burning (Butric Acid? to be used in 6 potency read the notes in the previous page).
Sul.Acid	Sour eructations, sets teeth on edge (Robinea) craving for alcohol. Relaxed feeling in stomach. Averse to smell of Coffee. Sour vomiting, coldness of stomach relieved by warm applications.

Continued...

HAEMATMESIS – (Remedies)	
Acid Sulph	Indicated in an aphthous condition of the mouth and esophagus with gastralgia, acidity of the stomach, and a sensation of tremor all over the body, with vomiting of dark blood. The stools consist of small black lumps mixed with blood. In this connection Acetic acid should also be remembered
Aconite	In acute cases attended with fear, restlessness, fever etc.
Arnica	This may be of service in cases of traumatism
Crotalus horr.	There is a rapid degeneration of the blood to such an extent that there are haemorrhages from any oral tissues. Lachesis should in connection with Crotalus.
Ergeron	The haemorrhages are bright red. There is violent retching and burning in the stomach, with vomiting of blood, and sharp cutting pains in the epigastric region every few minutes followed by a dull pain.
Hydrastis	This remedy has a most decided action in many of these cases, especially when there is a history of catarrhal affection, with discharges that are thick, white and tenacious, or yellow green and bloody. There is usually a history of gastric catarrh and persistent constipation. The second decimal trituration of Hydrsastine, Hydrchlorte is highly efficient.
Hamamelis	**Has been termed the Aconite of the venous system.** It should be remembered in these cases in which there is more or less of a general venous congestion, varicosities and a general tendency to venous haemorrhages.
Ipecac	Associated with nausea. The face is pale and the body rather cool. The blood is bright red, it has but little influence in those cases in which there is degeneration of the blood.
Millefolium	Should be studied in those cases in which the hemorrhage is more active than that of Hamamelis. There is excessive palpitation of the heart with malaise and weakness.

Phosphorous	Indicated in the tall, slender patient with fair skin, sanguine temperament and sensitive disposition who complains of a sensation of weakness and emptiness in the abdomen. There is frequently portal congestion and such degenerations as lead to haemorrhages.
Terebinthinam	This remedy in the **lower potency** is highly serviceable and especially if the hemorrhage is dependent upon a pathological condition of the stomach
Trillium	Copious hemorrhages and they are either active or passive and are usually of bright red blood. The patient has a disgust for everything except cold water. There are pains and cramps in the region of the stomach and vomiting of blood

CHAPTER – 8

TREATMENT OF OTHER PARTS OF ABDOMEN AND LIVER

Abdomen consists, Stomach (*the complaints thereof with remedies are already* **submitted earlier**) duodenum, small intestine, large intestine, spleen, lever and gall-bladder, pancreas, kidneys with the ureters, bladder, uterus in case of ladies. All these are covered with a serous membrane called peritoneum. Therefore, there can be ailment in any of these organs and the pain referred by the patient can be of any part of the organ and cannot be construed that all pains in abdomen pertain only to stomach.

Hence, one should carefully examine the location of pain so as to pin point the part of the organ ailing. It is also suggested that the available latest pathological reports, if any, are to be studied for which one should attain the minimum knowledge of reading these pathological reports so as to pin point the part of the abdomen ailing as it can help in selecting an appropriate remedy. The reasons of pain may be as under.

PAIN

The causes of abdominal pain are many. Its importance and significance demand the physician for an early and a most thorough through examination, to clearly understand interpretation. The old adage that an abdominal is the cry of hungry nerve for food, or an appeal for a sleeping potion, is no longer tenable, and it demands an explanation in the light of pathological anatomy of chemistry. The place of pain and the clinical history of lesion varies, in some cases it indicates the advent of the lesion, while in other cases is only present at the close.

When called to a case in which abdominal pain is present, the physician should secure as complete a clinical history as possible, obtaining all information regarding what preceded, accompanied or followed the advent of the pain. He should determine the cause of the pain and avoid the administration of opiates, which dulls his power of observation more than it does the patient's pain. The effect of the pain upon the patient should be observed, his facial expression, pulse, temperature, attitude and mental condition, as well as changes produced in the abdomen, as tenderness, muscular rigidity, distension or change of contour.

The site of the initial pain while not always trustworthy from a diagnostic standpoint, yet is frequently of service, and is decidedly of more service than the diffused pain which occurs later. In certain cases the pain is at first diffused and later becomes localised.

One of the most frequent causes of abdominal pain is an inflamed appendix. The pain at first is frequently referred to the epigastric or umbilical region and is diffused, while it becomes localized in the appendiceal region, and is associated with tenderness, muscular rigidity and vomiting. The pulse and temperature are variable and may be misleading. In certain cases there is no pain till the peritoneal coat is reached by the pathological process, when the pain appears suddenly it is intense and agonizing in character.

It should be borne in mind that severe pain in the right inguinal region may be dependent upon an infected gall-bladder, a floating kidney an occluded intestine, a ruptured extra-uterine gestation sac, a pleurisy, a specific salpingitis or a specific prostatitis.

In chronic appendicitis there is a history of repeated attacks while in perforating appendicitis the pain is agonizing and is followed by shock, normal or subnormal temperature, a rapid pulse, extreme rigidity of the abdominal wall, meteorism, and the pain subsides till the development of a more general peritonitis.

In gangrenous appendicitis the pain is intense, with extreme muscular rigidity, tenderness, rapid pulse, fever and anxiety. In all cases of appendicitis, the sudden subsidence of abdominal pain should be considered grave, as indicating a perforation.

ACUTE INTESTINAL CATARRHA

Synonym: Acute diarrhea, acute catarrhal enteritis, ileo cholitis

This is an inflammation of the mucous membranes of small intestine and in some cases the upper portion of the colon.

AETIOLOGY: The most frequent cause is dietetic error that results in irritation of the intestinal mucous membrane, as the ingestion of decomposed foods and drinks, unripe fruits or vegetables, fermented drinks, putrid water or food that is insufficiently masticated or is indigestible. Certain articles of diet that may be well borne by one may be an irritant to another and act as an exciting cause. It may result from certain irritant poisons, exposure to, or applications of cold. At times may be epidemic during the hot summer months, or during the autumn. This may be secondary to typhoid fever, measles, diabetes, malaria and certain constitutional and acute diseases.

SYMPTOMS:

These vary with the extent of the disease and the portion of the bowel involved. If the large bowel is involved, diarrhea is present. When the process confined to the small intestine, diarrhea may not be present, as the faecal matter acquires a consistency in the healthy large intestine. There is usually colicky, abdominal pain, with a moderate gaseous distension of the abdomen, rumbling and gurgling noises and occasionally vomiting. The tongue is furred there is thirst, anorexia and scanty urine. The temperature is usually normal but may be slightly elevated (100.5 F)

When the duodenum alone is involved there is constipation with a slight pain and tenderness that are indefinite. Usually there is nausea and vomiting and gastric distress (gastro duodenitis). In this condition there is also slight jaundice, but the symptoms are indefinite.

When the colon is involved there is more pain and diarrhea with tenderness along the course of the colon. The stools are soup-like and contain large quantities of mucus. If the rectum is involved there is severe pain and tenesmus and large quantities of mucus and pus.

CHRONIC INTESTINAL CATARRH

Synonyms: Chronic diarrhea, chronic enteritis

Pathology: Mucous membrane, the seat of lesion, may be of a brownish red or grayish red appearance. The brownish haemoglobin may be transformed into a black melanin and the mucous membrane present a mottled appearance. Secretions are increased and the mucous membrane is covered with clear or turbid mucus. The lymph follicles are enlarged. Mucous membrane is thickened as a result of the hyperplasia of the connective tissue and often the muscular layer and the mucosa are involved in the hyperplasia and thickening. In some cases atrophy takes place and an atrophic intestinal catarrh results. In other cases a disintegration of the lymph follicles takes place, follicular intestinal ulcerating ensues or a destruction of the mucosa takes place and catarrhal ulceration of the mucous membrane results.

Symptoms: The main symptom is alteration in the stools, which are frequent and of diminished consistency. In some cases there is abundant mucus which may envelop the feacal matter if in the large intestine and in the small intestine they are mixed. Constipation and diarrhea may alternate. Stools may contain a large amount of undigested material. Swollen sago-like granules are present in the stool. Blood may be observed in the stool. There is usually more or less rumbling and distension of the abdomen with flatus, while abdominal pain and tormina may be severe. Stools may contain undigested particles of food. The nutrition of the patient suffers. He becomes emaciated and acquires a greyish sallow appearance, becomes hypochondrical, develops delusions, fears that he will become insane, doubts of his mental and physical condition. He is apt to be annoyed with vertigo, which is often produced or aggravated voluntarily by pressure upon the abdomen. There is also palpitation of heart and asthamatic attacks. The appetite is variable and thirst is increased. Urine is of a dark colour and precipitates reddish granular sediment of urates. It contains indican.

CHRONIC INTESTINAL CATARRH (Remedies)	
Ars. Alb.	When there are present the restlessness with anguish and a desire to constantly change the position, together with the violent unquenchable, burning thirst for small quantities of water at frequent intervals. There is often nausea and vomiting immediately after eating or drinking. If the stools are watery, they are very offensive and usually without pain, while if they are mucous, they are usually offensive.
Arg. Nit.	Indicated following dysentery and when a chronic condition of ulceration remains. The patient is greatly emaciated. There is a tremulous weakness with debility and vertigo. Flatulent colic with loud eructations, at times an ineffectual effort to eructate which causes strangling. Stools vary in colour, but often consist of green mucous like chopped spinach expelled forcibly with much spluttering. These patients are fond of sweets but are aggravated by them.
CHRONIC INTESTINAL CATARRH (Remedies)	
Calc. Carb	In the selection of this remedy the type of the patient and the general symptoms must be taken carefully. Patient is fat (false plethora). There are profuse sweats about the head when sleeping, especially on the back of the head. Feet are constantly cold and damp. The abdomen is large and distended. Stomach is irritable and there is sour vomiting.

Continued...

Cinchona	Should be compared carefully with Carbo veg. They are also worse after a meal. The stools show partially digested food, are painless and are attended with much flatulence. There is marked distension of the abdomen, which is temporarily relieved by belching.
Gambogia	Indicated when there is a history of a continued looseness of bowels or alternate constipation and diarrhea. The stool is thin and yellow and comes out all at once with a simple, somewhat prolonged effort, which is followed by sensation of great relief, as though an irritating substance has been removed from the intestine. The anus feels sore and burnt.
Geranium Maculatum	Should be studied in cases where there are abnormal discharges from the mucous surfaces after the inflammation has subsided. There is a constant desire to go to stool, with inability to pass the least feacal matter. One to five drops of tincture (Q) or in 3rd potency should be given every three hours.
Merc Cor	When there is present a constant & severe tenesmus and when stools contain much blood and pus. The abdomen is distended and painful.
Natrum sulph	Has a decided action in controlling morning diarrhea that appears later than that of Sulphur. Stools are of a yellowish-green colour and gushing in character. Before the stool there is rumbling in the abdomen and colic, with a profuse emission of flatus accompanying the stool, giving relief from the colic. There are stitches in the hepatic region, and the liver is tender to pressure.
Rhatanhia	Has proven of service in some of these cases, when associated with fissures and ulcers of the anus.

Sulphur	This remedy is frequently indicated in acute as well as chronic cases. The apparently indicted remedy does not afford the desired relief, or its effect is but transient. The diarrhea is worse during the morning and frequently drives the patient out of bed early. The evacuations are painless, the odour of the stools follows him as though he had soiled his linen and there is an offensive odour of the body despite frequent washing. The patient shows excessive prostration, becomes emaciated rapidly, and he is apt to be excoriated about the anus.

CHOLERA INFANTUM

Synonym: Acute milk infection.

AetiologySymptoms:

At times with diarrheal movements of the bowels, but usually: It is believed that this is a toxic condition produced by the absorption from the intestinal canal of the toxic fermentation of food, especially impure milk. It occurs moist frequently during the months of July and August, and among infants living under defective hygienic conditions, and frequently with an improper diet. There is a brief period during which child is restless and appears to have some abdominal distress. The temperature rises, the child begins to vomit and this is soon followed by purging. Vomiting is nearly continuous and consists at first of the contents of the stomach, then bile stained mucus and finally serous fluid. The evacuations from the bowels follows similar course, become copious, fluid, alkaline in reaction and have a musty odour. The microscope shows them to consist of epithelial debris, round cells and bacteria. The discharge contain little or through no feacal material, and pass through the diaper. There is not much pain, and while the surface of the body and extremities feels cold to the hand, the rectal temperature is usually from 103 to 105 F. The child is thirsty, but all fluid taken into the stomach is speedily rejected. It loses strength and weight. The face becomes of an ashy hue, eyes are sunken and pinched. The pulse is quick and weak, and intermittent, while urine is scanty and may be suppressed. The restlessness which characterises the early stages is replaced by apathy, which is followed later by a hydrocephloid state, when the head is drawn backward and may be moved from side to side. The pupils are sluggish and may be unequal. The abdomen is retracted and the respirations are irregular. At the end approaches the child becomes more comatose and often passes into a convulsion which closes the scene. Ocasionally hyperpyrexia is present before death. In some cases the process is so rapid that collapse and death take place within twenty-four hours. In those cases that recover the vomiting ceases, stools gradually return to normal feacal character, character of the pulse improves, the restlessness abates, convalescens slow and relapses are not uncommon.

Treatment:

When the disturbance appears, the stomach should be given a rest. If breast fed, the period between the feedings should be prolonged, or the child should not be not be allowed to remain so long at the breast as usual. If the child fed on artificial food, it should be withheld for from twelve to twenty-four hours. During this period water may be given and at the end of this period albumen water or barley water may be used for twenty-four hours. If the food the child has been taking before the attack has agreed, it may be gradually resumed, but diminished in amount and at lengthened periods between the feedings. If the intestines show much involvement in the process they should be cleaned out by a high injection or by other means. If the intestines show much involvement in the process they should be cleaned out by a high injection or by other means. If the vomiting and diarrhea have been such that there has been great loss of fluid, large quantities of water should be given, high enemata of normal salt solutions or hypodermoclysters. For an infant, a pint and a half may be used five or six times a day. High fever should be treated by hydrotherapy, the child being bathed every hour or two.

Low temperature should be avoided. The water should be employed but a few degrees below the rectal temperature of the patient. The patient should be kept warm by wrapping in warm flannels surrounded by warm bottles. Food should be given hot. An excellent stimulant for many of these cases consists in a mustard bath. One tablespoonful of mustard should be put in a bag made of loose cloth; this should be put into the bath tub at the far end from the child. The child should be kept in the bath till reaction sets in upon the arm of the attendant who is holding the child. No reaction on the part of the child from such a bath is an unfavourable condition. At times the eyes require a wash of boric acid solution. If the eyelids remain open, as they do at times, a piece of fine lint saturated with boric acid should be kept over the eyes. The disease is at times followed by cholera typhoid; this requires care in diet, stimulants, hydrotherapy and remedies.

CHOLERA INFANTUM (Remedies)	
Aconite	Indicated in the early stages when the child is restless, the pulse is feeble, then there is cold sweat, motor and sensory paralysis, vomiting and purging, and even convulsions. In spite of the cold sweat, the rectal temperature will be found high.
Ars alb.	Indicated when there is extreme restlessness and prostration with unquenchable thirst for small quantities of water. The face is pale and cadaveric and the skin is cold. There is frequent vomiting and purging. The stools are frequent, offensive and watery.
Cup Ars.	Indicated when the stools are watery and serous and may be of greenish colour. There is usually pain in the abdomen, and cramping in the extremities.
Camphor	When there is an early and sudden collapse, with cold sweat on the face and a cold blue surface. The voice is weak and hoarse and the infant is almost unconscious. The stools are painless.

Continued...

Euphorbia corrollata	Is indicated when there is sudden and profuse vomiting, first the contents of the stomach, while later it is a rice water material. There is a copious water diarrhoea, which alternates with the vomiting. There are cramps in the intestines, with anxiety faintness and exhaustion.
Secale cor.	Should be remembered when the acuteness of the attack has passed. The stools are watery and profuse, and are attended with great prostration, coldness of the surface of the body and dislike of being covered.
Veratrum alb.	There is vomiting and purging. The stools are profuse, like rice water, and a cold sweat, especially upon the forehead. The child is greatly exhausted and even in a state of collapse. There are cramps in the extremities.
Zincum met.	Remembered late in the attack, when the features are sunken and the patient is in a state of collapse. The eyes remain open, the fontanelles are sunken and there is deficient nerve power. The temperature is abnormal and there is an absence of reaction.

CHOLERA MORBUS

Synonym: Cholera nostras

Aetiology:

It occurs in those of all ages, is most frequent during the summer months and is favoured by the eating of unripe vegetables and fruits, drinking ice water, iced beverages, partaking of ice cream, exposure to wet and cold and to unhygienic surroundings.

Symptoms:

These appear suddenly. The patient is taken with severe abdominal pains and vomiting. The vomited material may contain partially digested food, which later becomes mixed with bile and mucus. While the vomiting is in progress the abdominal pains become intense. The stools soon lose their feacal character and become serous, not unlike the "rice water", discharge of Asiatic cholera. There is coldness of the extremities and cold perspiration appears on the forehead. The rectal temperature shows an elevation from one to seven degrees. The pulse is feeble and rapid, the face pale, pinched and cyanotic. The urine is high coloured and may contain albumin, is scanty and in severe cases anuria (absence of urine) may be present. The thirst is extreme. There are cramps of the extremities and there is tenderness over the colon.

Treatment:

The patient should remain in bed, all gastric and intestinal discharges should be removed from the room at once. **No food should be administered during the first twenty four hours.** *The patient should not take much fluid during this time, even if desire to do so is pronounced,* as it increases the amount of fluid in the intestinal tract and increases the vomiting and diarrhoea. To control the thirst, small pieces of ice may be held in the mouth, or small amounts of weak cold tea without sugar or cold oat meal water may be allowed.

As the symptoms, half milk may be allowed. Gradually boiled rice or mik toast may be added. The second day, if the vomiting and diarrhoea have ceased, the diet may be increased, and soft boiled or poached eggs, raw oysters, scraped beef and crackers, toast, or well boiled rice may be allowed. If the condition has **persisted** for several days, greater **care must be exercised in the care of the diet.** When the pain is severe, hot applications to the epigastrium, or over the right pneumogastric nerve in the side of the neck, are of service. Patients who are subject to these attacks, as a result of exposure, should wear a flannel bandage over the abdomen. Where dehydration takes place, saline hypodermoclysters are of service.

CHOLERA MORBUS: (Remedies)	
Ars. alb.	Indicated in cases characterized by sudden and extreme prostration and collapse. Patient complains of severe burning distress in the region of the stomach. There is a violent thirst for frequent but small quantities of water, which is immediately thrown up. There is great dyspnoea and with it an inexpressible anguish, weakened pulse, and a constant desire to move. The vomiting is violent, and is repeated as soon as the slightest material enters the stomach. The evacuations of the bowels are frequent and are attended by excoriations of the skin and mucous membrane about the anus. The stools are dark, acrid and putrid, and cause a sensation of burning of the anus. There is coldness of the extremities, with exhaustion and trembling of the whole body.
Ant. Crud.	Should be studied in cases characterized by a milk – white tongue and a history of the overloading of the stomach. There is no thirst. The vomiting continues after the nausea has ceased. Stools while watery contain hard lumps of feacal material. The attack may have been caused by acids, overheating, cold bathing, cold food, from summer heat or debauch. Before and during the stool there are cutting pains in the rectum, while following the stools there is a sensation as though the anus was excoriated.
Cup. Met	Indicated when there are violent cramps and spasms attending the attack. The cramps are mostly noticeable in the flexor muscles so that they are drawn up into visible knots. The patient is restless, tosses about and is in constant uneasiness. The eyes are sunken and have blue rings about them, there is an intense coldness and blueness of the surface, with long continued general cold sweat, and great prostration. There is a deathly sensation, with nausea and vomiting of a greenish water, which is attended by a copious greenish diarrhoea and violent pain in the bowels

China	Indicated in cases that have not yielded promptly to treatment. The patient complains of great weakness, rapid exhaustion and emaciation, as a result of the prolonged low of fluids. The stools vary in appearance. They are more frequent after meals and at night. There is tympanitis with emissions of large quantities of flatus; and evacuations which afford temporary relief.
Croton	When the stool is yellow and watery in character, is expelled suddenly, "coming out like a shot" and there is aggravation from food, drink, or while nursing.
Dioscorea	Should be remembered when accompanying the nausea and vomiting, there is violent twisting colic which occurs in regular proxims with remissions. There are severe darting, cutting pains in the sacral region and bowels, which radiate upwards and downwards till whole body, even the fingers and toes, are involved in the spasms, which cause the patient to shriek. The patient finds relief by standing and bending backward.
Elateriaum	Indicated for the olive-green, frequent, copious discharge that follow exposure after exertion
Gambogia	Should be remembered when the evacuation comes out all at once with a single, somewhat prolonged effort. This is followed by a sensation as though some irritating substance had been removed from the bowel
Ipecacuanha	Indicated when there is continuous nausea. It is indicated in the early history of the case and often requires another remedy to complete the cure. With the continuous nausea and vomiting the tongue is clean, there is no thirst and the patient loathes food. The stool consists of green mucus, "as green as grass". The face is pale the pupils are dilated, there is a cold upon the forehead and there are blue rings about the eyes.
Podophyllum	For the painless form when the stools appears to drain the patient

Continued...

MUCUS COLITIS

Synonyms: Mucus enteritis, Membraneous colitis

Pathology:

On inspection the mucosa is found evidently thickened, changed in colour and covered with a rather tenacious mucus. The connective tissue is increased due to the inflammatory process. The lymphatic follicles are increased in size, sub-mucosa is increased in thickness and more or less vascular engorgement is noticed. In long drawn out cases hypertrophy or atrophy of the intestinal walls may result and occasionally a peculiar blood pigmentation is observed. Ulceration of the intestinal walls may result either as a simple solution of continuity or from a necrotic process. As a sequel to such process, submucous abscess may result followed by partial adhesions and serious peritoneal and abdominal complications. The ulcerative process may be followed by cicatrisation and resulting narrowing of the lumen of the bowel.

The microscope shows the stools top consist of feacal matter, mucus, epithelial and pus cells, and various micro-organisms. When the stools are washed the residue often looks like boiled sago grains. The mucous may separate from the wall of the intestine without leaving any lesion.

Symptoms:

As a class these patients are thin, pale, poorly nourished & anaemic. They are poor eaters and eliminate one article of food after another from their diet which they believe has distressed them. They suffer from severe occipital headaches and periods of mental depression. The nervous exhibition vary in character and there may be present all forms of the hysterical stigamata. The attack may develop abruptly or insidiously. If developed abruptly, colic like abdominal pains predominate and may be very severe. They are usually most severe in the epigastrium, in the left iliac fossa; occasionally the entire abdominal area is affected. The pain may extend to the bladder, genitals and even radiate to the legs, especially the left, accompanied by considerable tenesmus. While this false membrane of mucous is forming the symptoms are aggravated but there is a cessation of pain for a period following its separation and passage. The pains may return several times a day, or may occur once a week or a month. Preceding the attack there is anorexia, constipation, a general nervous state and great mental depression. A condition of constipation or alternate diarrhoea may be present. The pulse rate is not much disturbed and elevation of temperature is very rare. In less acute cases the stools are hard, the mucus is seen in large flakes or strings winding about the stool.

MUCUS COLITIS – (Remedies)	
Ant. Crud.	This remedy produces an excessive amount of mucus upon the intestinal mucous membrane. The digestion is interfered with and there is fermentation and belching. There is alternately constipation and diarrhoea. The stools are often lumpy and accompanied with large quantities of mucus. The diarrhoea is aggravated by acid drinks, cold bathing, and overheating. The great characteristic is the thick, white coating on the tongue.
Asarum Eur.	Its proving has developed many symptoms similar to this condition and has been a means of relief in several cases. The patient is nervous, of an excitable or melancholic mood and the least noise is unbearable. There is pain in the left side of the abdomen, that extends to the back in the region of descending colon, attended with large quantities of stringy mucus from the bowel that may form a large part of the stool. When the bowels become constipated there is headache.

Continued...

Aur.Nat.Mur (Gold & Sodium Chloride 2x)	Indicated in the neurotic cases where there is severe gastro-enteritis attended with convulsions, insomnia constipation, and an increased secretion of mucus from the intestinal glands. There is dyspepsia with pain in the region or the descending colon. The tongue is red and glazed. There is anorexia with extreme tenderness in the epigastric region. The patient is depressed and melancholy
Colocynath	The pain is severe, causing the patient to struggle. It is griping, cutting or squeezing in character, and causes the sufferer to bend double. There is relief from hard pressure and aggravation from eating and drinking
Dioscorea	There are griping pains in the abdomen which come at regular intervals, and are as though the intestines were grasped by a powerful hand. Patient is made worse by lying down, bending forward and is relieved by standing up/ bending backward
Graphites	Stools are hard, lumpy and are accompanied by discharges of shreds of mucus. There is a sensation of weight and uneasiness in the abdomen.
Hydrastis	Produces a condition similar to mucous colitis. The patient is debilitated and suffers from marked derangement of the gastric and hepatic functions. The tongue is broad and shows the imprint of teeth. There are catarrhal discharges which are thick, yellow and stringy
Mag Phos.	To relieve the pains in thin, dark, emaciated individuals with highly developed organisms. The pains are sharp and cutting, coming & going, causing the patient to bend double. They are relieved by heat, by rubbing and by hard pressure.
Merc.Sol/Cor	The patient cannot lie on right side; bitter taste; more thirst and hunger; continual chilliness; yellow colour of the skin and eye; fullness and tenderness across the epigastrium and hypochondria; on walking bowels shake as if loose; slimy, bloody stools, preceded by anxiety, trembling, faint ness.

Nux. vom	Irritable patient, with dark hair and bilious temperament, who are nervous, melancholic, and oversensitive to external impressions, and to whom trifling ailments are unbearable. There is frequent unsuccessful desire to pass small quantities of feaces.
Oxalic acid:	Stomach sensitive; slightest touch causes excoriating pains; colic about the navel, as if bruised, with stitches and difficult emission of flatulence, < on moving > when at rest; constant involuntary stools; stools of mucus and blood.
Podophyllum	Enteritis affecting the jejunum and ilium; fullness in right hypochondrium, with flatulence, pain and soreness; frequent but transsient abdominal pains, with sensation of heat there; alternate constipation an diarrhoea.
Vertrum alb.	Cold feeling in stomach an abdomen; cold sweat; cold extremeties; pinche face; nausea with sensation of fainting, with violent thirst; painful retraction of abdomen during vomit ing also burning as from hot coals in abdomen, which is very sensitive; intestinal catarrh, coming on suddenly at night, in summer, stools watery, greenish, mixed with flakes.

GIARDIASIS: PROTOZOAL LIKE THAT OF E. HYSTOLICA (AMOEBIASIS) –

Symptoms:

Diarrhoea, anoxeria (loss of appetite) – Pain in abdomen, flatulence, Indigestion, constipation and other symptoms – Here the flatulency, distension of abdomen and acidity are more prominent than in **Amoebiasis** – Symptoms observed in the patients, percentage-wise, are as under:

Amoebiasis

Symptoms observed are as under:

SYMPTOMS	% of Patients
Pain in abdomen	99
Anorexia (Loss of appetite)	73
Loose motions – chronic	71
Acute	63
Pallor	56
Distention of Abdomen	52
Indigestion	50
Repeated attacks of cough	48
Flatulence	44
Tenesmus	35
Fever	30
Voracious appetite	27
Vomiting	27
Constipation	21
Prolapsed rectum	19
Pica	19
Nausea	12
Not growing well	11
Urgency of defecation	09
Irritability	06
Urticaria	03
Depigmented patches over the face	02
A-symptomatic	01

AMOEBIASIS

Synonyms: Fux, Bloody flux

Varieties: Catarrhal, Amebic or Tropical,. Chronic: This disease is protozoa infection. These protozoa are Entiamoeba Histolytica. This infection takes place either by house fly which infect the food, or drinking water which may be contaminated by these protozoa, where there is a leakage from the drainage pipes.

Having gained entrance through the infected food stuffs into the digestive canal of a susceptible person. It passes unaltered through the stomach and towards the caecium. In this alkaline media of the caecium these protozoa take encystic form and throws out a single amoeba containing four neucli and again it divides into eight neucli. Tropozites are liberated from encystic stage. These are the active forms of the protozoa. They enter through crypts of the liberthium and penetrate directly through the columnar epithelium of the mucous membrane of the gut by their amoboid movement and by destroying the tissue by producing proteolytic ferment. By this continuous lyses they burrow into the deeper tissues and lodge in the sub mucus membrane. They colonise there and multiply and go on destroying the tissues and gradually recede from dead tissue towards the margin of healthy tissue in the large gut producing deep ulcerations with much of fibrosis, tracing undermined flask shaped edges. So it produces daily eight to ten loose motions with mucous, blood and feacus. There will not be much cellular tissue in the stool. The protozoa produce Acid secretions in the intestines and increase the acid and fermentation and thereby flatulency thereat. These acute symptoms continue for some days or month and remissions follow. Sometimes rectum is also involved in the severe ulceration producing tenesmus, straining and with streaks of mucus, dark stool with a penetrating odour.

As it becomes there, there will be definite distension over caecium with abdominal tenderness where it may stimulate appendicitis with pain at M burney's point with vomiting at times. Sometimes reflex stimulation of the stomach gives out the symptoms resembling the gastric ulcer whenever the transverse colon is affected, with sound eructations and vomiting which relieve pain.

These tropzoites by embolic phenomena are carried through portal vein to the liver from intestine and causes inflammation of the liver and even leads to abscess. Especially this abscess is seen in the posterior superior surface of the right lobe of the liver and it contains sloughed liver tissue and blood. The colour of this blood is chocolate brown and it is otherwise said to be ANCHORY SAUCE. This produces pain in the right hypochondriac region, weight and fullness with pain shooting towards the right shoulder. The appetite is poor, easy satiety and bloating of the abdomen with discomfort and intolerance of fatty food with flatulency, dyspepsia. Later there will be swinging temperature sweating, running down conditions with debility and easy fatigue and always wants to take rest. Dreads to undertake any new task, depressed, cannot concentrate on anything, dull melancholic, forgetful, asthenic, with disquamation of the skin and atrophy of the nails. Most of the people due to this get debility, palpation and dull pains in the precordial region and sort of cardiac irritability where the person is always conscious of his heart and he will get thoughts of suicide. On examination, the liver is palpable, tender and the dullness extends upwards. If the abscess is high enough, pushes the diaphragm upwards and causes the collapse of the base of the right lung with a diminished movement of the right base.

Sometimes this abscess bursts into the right lungs and causes by abscess, or emphymia, if it rupture into the pleura. If the abscess is on the left lobe of the liver it may also bursts into the stomach; it may cause peritonitis. The vegetative forms of the active stage of the disease enter into the lungs and produce symptoms mimicking Tuberculosis. That is, evening rise of temperature, cough, running down condition and thick yellowish expectoration. The X – ray shows a definite patch in the affected area of the lung making the diagnosis confused. Most of the doctors think that it is Tuberculosis and start anti-tubercular treatment.

If these emboli travel and lodge in the brain they form abscess of the brain. It also produces proliferative granular masses on the skin bear the visceral lesions called amoebiasis cutis. But it is a naked and admitted fact that susceptibility counts much. The protozoa or bacteria cannot grow unless there is susceptibility. We say these protozoa or bacteria are ultimates of the disease. We believe that inherited chronic miasm like Psora, Sycosis and Syphilis either individually or by combination give such a kind of susceptibility so that one can attract diseases. By seeing these above said chronic destructions strongly believe that this disease is **due to combination of Psora and Syphilis and is seen on the background of tubercular diathesis.**

AMOEBIASIS – TREAMENT

The important thing lies with homoeopathy is individualizing the patient. **We are having medicines for patients and not for the disease.** We must gather the symptoms from the patients, like modalities, uncommon, peculiar characteristics sensations, desires and aversions and also concomitants for prescription: As under:

Pain abdomen > bending backwards	Dioscorea
Pain abdomen > by bending double with hot fomentation	Colocynth, Mag Phos
With each and every griping pain rushing to stool	Nux vom
Excessive hunger with easy satiety,dyspepsia with flatulency	Lycopodium < 4 t0 8 p.m.
Desire for sugar it causes loose motion with anticipation neurosis	Arg. Nit
Sensation as if anus is wide open	Phosphorous
Never get done feeling with tenesmus <night	Merc.sol
Dyspnoea, cough> by drinking cold water	Causticum
Dyspnoea, cough > by eating	Spongia
Sweetish taste of the sputum	Stannum
As a specific remedy towards: E.Hystolica	KURCHI Q– 5–6 drops in water @ 8 a.m

Continued...

AMOEBIASIS – – (Remedies)	
Aloes	Is found occasionally indicated when abdomen is tender to pressure and there is sensation as though it was greatly distended. The stools are scanty, watery, bloody, jelly like, and are attended with severe tenesmus which forces the hemorriodal vessels out. They are large, tender, but relieved by cold applications.
Baptisia	It should be studied that assumes typhoid type. The stools may consist of pure blood or they may be dark, thin, and feacal in character. Whatever the character of the stool, it is **horribly offensive.** There is colic beforehand during the stool, and relief of it after stool, while the tenesmus is during and following the stool. The patient's face is dark red, and presents a besotted look. The tongue has a yellow brown coating in the centre with red, shining edges. The patient complains of a bruised sore feeling over the whole body which causes restlessness. The patient frequently complains of not being able to sleep on account of a sensation as though the body were scattered about the bed, and cause him to toss about.
Colocynth	Should be remembered when there are severe agonizing pains in the abdomen, with intense cutting, squeezing pains which cause the patient to bend double. The pain is relieved by pressure and bending double and is made worse by eating and drinking. The stools are at first watery and mucous, then bilious, and later bloody.
Ipecac	It is indicated when the usual symptoms are intensified and the strength of the patient is failing. There is great tenesmus, the stools are dark green or frothy like molasses, and may contain blood.
Merc.Sol or Vivus	One of these preparations should be studied in those cases of diarrhoea where there is tendency to dysentery. It is useful in the dysentery of children and in cases where there is no great amount of blood and less pain than that which characterizes the Corrosives.

Mag, Sulph 1X	Is indicated when the stools are copious and watery. There is rumbling and distension of the abdomen. The cause of the attack is usually a sudden change of the temperature.
Podophylium	There is present a stool consisting of glairy blood with violent tenesmus, soon leads to prolapsus of the rectum.
Rheum	Indicated at the onset of the attack and again at the close, where there is cutting pain and rumbling in the bowels. The stools are feacal, soft, have strong, sour odor and contain but little mucus. One drop of the tincture every two hours is of service.

Use Kurchi Q or Chaparo Amargosa Q or Aegal Mar Q – depending upon symptoms, daily ¾ drops in one ounce water @ 8 AM and 8 PM with other indicated remedies as above used for 2 or three days for Amoebiasis or Giardiasis till complete relief is there. **Intermittently use Nux Vom 30 in Amoebiasis or Giardiasis**

DIARRHOEA: Remedies	
Aloes	Rumbling in abdomen – gushing stools
Ars.Alb.	Cold drinks or food poisoning with vomiting
Camphor	Cold body with and almost collapse stage
Nu Vom	Acid smelling stools, late dinners, contaminated food, due to indigestion and sedentary life style
Nat.Mur	Summer Diarrhoea
Podophyllum	Summer diarrhoea
Veratrum Alb.	Choleric symptoms prominent with great weakness an coldness of the body
Also study Croton Tig., Jatropia, Cambhogia	

DYSENTERY

Enforce recumbent position in bed, even for a stool; keep towel under patient and let mucous or bloody passages fall on toilet paper and keep your patient clean, lying on back or left side.

DYSENTERY REMEDIES	
Aconite	WHEN THE DAYS ARE WARM AND THE NIGHTS COOL Scanty, loose, frequent stools with tenesus; small brown, painful, at last bloody, or pure blood passes without faeces, rheumatic pains in head, nape of neck and shoulders, or violent chill, heat and unquenchable thirst, fear and restlessness.
Aloe	Aggravation by acids; SHOOTING OR BORING pains in the region of the navel, INCREASED BY PRESSURE; the lower part of the abdomen swollen and sensitive to pressure; the distension and movements in the abdomen are more in the LEFT SIDE and along the track of the colon, INCREASED AFTER FOOD; FAINTING WHILST AT STOOL OR AFTER; frequent stools of bloody water, bloody, jellylike mucus, involuntary while passing flatus, great repugnance to fresh air which, notwithst nding, ailments the suffering; hunger during the stool; cutting and pinching in the rectum and loins, heaviness, weariness and numbness in the thighs; with the stools escape large quantities of flatuis; wjen urinating urging to stool; sicknes of stomach andgreat prostration, constamt headache and some nausea; dryness of the mouth; thirst; discharge of a few drops of foul-smelling, bloody mucus, with violent tenesmus, which may continue after the dysentary.
Apis Mell	Chronic dysentery, frequent discharge of gelatinous mucous with slight tenesmus; general soreness of abdomen, especially over transverse and descending colon; more urging than actual pain, throbbing in rectum with sensation in anus as if it were stuffed full; rawness of anus; tongue dry, shining, white; urine frequent, profuse, or strangury; skin hot, dry, yet little thirst, disturbed sleep, with muttering. Infant ile dysentery with frequent, painless, bloody stools, < mornings; prolapsus ani.

Alstonia const.	Dysentery complicated with sy mptoms of malaria or caused by DRINKING SWAMP-WATER IMPREGNATED WITH DECAYING VEGETABLE MATTER.
Alumen	PUTRID DYSENTERY; violent pains going from rectum down the thighs; during stool dyspnoea, pains in rectum, tenesmus, after stool scarcely endurable pain (scirrhus in rectum).
Argentum nit.	Dysentric stools, consisting of masses of epithelial substance, connected by muco-lymph, red or green, shreddy, frequent, with seavering bearing down in the hypogastrium; CRAMP OF THE RECTUM; thin unshapely strips pass in masses, with burning, constriction and soreness in left side of the abdomen; advanced case of dysentery, with suspected ulceration.
Baptisia	Adynamic dysenteria, PROSTRATION MUCH MORE PROFOUND THAN THE LOSS OF BLOOD OR PAIN WOULD JUSTIFY, brown tongue, low fever, rigors, pain in limbs and small of back; stools small, all blood, not very dark, but thick; tenesmus; violent colicky pain in hypogastric region; ulcerative inflammation of lower part of bowels in hot weather or in the fall; rejects all solid food.
Bryonia	Ofen after Aconite, especially during hot summer and from taking cold drinks; the least motion of the body, raising the arms, even bending the toes, produces a disposition to stool.
Baryta Carb	Stools of a jellylike appearance, with blood and NO PAIN whatever; discharges every 15 or 20 minutes; round pinworms pass with the stool; dysentery after suppression of humid tetters; paleness and emaciation.

Continued...

Belladonna	TENESMUS so severe as to cause shuddering; cutting tearing pains; burning of anus; tongue dry, very red at the tip, or two white stripes on a red ground, urine profuse or suppressed; dry, hot skin or hot sweat; thirst, yet averse to drink starts in sleep; stupor; sensitiveness of the abdomen; constant pressure to the anus and genitals, as everything would be pushed out; pains of a consisting character, relieved by bending forward and by pressure.
Calcarea carb	Chronic dysentry; pressure or straining in rectum; constant desire for stool; heaviness and burning in lower portion of rectum; discharge of blood or bloody mucus from rectum.
Cantharis	Colic urging and pinching before stool; pressing pain in intestines and anus, extorting cries, with cutting and burning in anus during stool; tenesmus after stool, like scraping from intestines, with streaks of blood; passage of pure blood from anus and urethra; chilliness as though water were poured over one, with internal warmth; dryness of lips and thirst during pains and yet loathing of drinks; vesicles and cankers in mouth and throat; collapse, small pulse, coldness of hands and feet. TENESMUS ASSOCIATED WITH DYSURIA (Merc.cor).
Capscicum	DYSENNTERY IN MOIST WETHER. < from any current of air, even when warm; violent tenesmus of rectum and bladder at the same time (Merc.or.); bloody, mucous, shaggy stools, > to night. Cutting, flatulent colic, twisting pains about navel, before stool, cutting and twisting, tenesmus, during stool, tenesmus, burning at anus, drawing pains in back, after stool. Thirst, but drinking causes shuddering; stool after drinking; suits stout, collapse; pulse weak and intermittent, cold breath.
Carbo veg.	Frequently involuntary stools of PUTRID CADAVEROUS ODOR; burning pains deep in abdomen, usually in one or other bend of the colon, abdomen tympanatic with much putrid flatus; feaces escape with flatus; collapse; pulse weak and intermittent, cold breath.

Carbolic acid	Bloody and mucous discharge, appearing like scraping of mucous membrane (Canth.); tenesmus; tenderness over transverse colon; tongue dry and coated with thick, yellow fur, great thirst and high fever.
Chamomilla	After Aconite. Mental symptoms decide.
China	DYSENTRY IN MARSHY DISTRICTS; with intermittent symptoms or when Ars. and Carb.v. fail to remove the putrid symptoms, stools become gradually more and more watery, pale, pinkish, with rapid emaciation, < after eating and drinking, at night; cold hands and feet.
Cistus Canad	CHRONIC DYSENTERY; desire for acid food and fruit, but they cause pain and cold feeling in stomach, with increase of stools.
Cornus circinata	Dysentery with INACTIVITY OF THE LIVER; stools dark, bilious, very offensive, bearing down pains in rectum and bowels, with urgent desire to go to stool; ulceration of mucous membrane of rectum.
Colchicum	Very painful urging to stool, at first only a little faeces pass, afterwards transperant, gelatinous and very membranous mucus, with some relief of pain in abdomen; water, jellylike mucus passes from anus with violent spasm in sphincter; bloody stools, with scrapings from intestines and prostration of anus; forcing, pressing pain in rectum with frequent scanty discharge; long-lasting agonizing pain in rectum and anus after stool, causing screams and crying, BLOODY STOOL, WITH DEATHLY NAUSEA FROM SMELLING COOKING, great weaknes and exhaustion as after exertion, cannot move head from pillow without help; keeps legs bent on abdomen to avoid distress when straightening them out; frequent shuddering down the back; cramps in calves of legs; burning or icy coldness of stomach. AUTUMNAL DYSENTERY.

Continued...

Colocynthis	Dysentric diarrhoea, < after least food or drink, with compressive, griping pains, commencing at navel and pasing down to rectum; stools bloody, full of mucus, passing every half hour, with great straining and burning of anus, TEMPORATILY CEASING AFTER STOOL AND BY WARMTH IN BED; weakness, paleness and prostration after stool; colicky cutting and squeezing pains > by bending forward and accompanied by disposition to stool; burning along urethra during stool; chills proceeding from abdomen.
Conium	CHRONIC DYSENTERY, slime mixed with greenish substances and containing bloody specks, stools small, offensive, with tenesmus and discharge of flatus during the passage, followed by weak, trembling feeling; no pain, < at night; appetite poor, craving for salt things.
Crotalus	Dysentery of septic origin, from foul water, food, etc., excessive flow of dark fluid blood or involuntary ercuations; great debility and faintness.
Cubeba	Discharges colourles, transparent mucus mixed with bright blood and PLENTIFULLY INTERSPERSED WITH SHINING WHIT E BODIES THE SHAPE OF RICE KERNELS, before stool severe griping in bowels with backache, uring stool the same urging to stool and to micturate, after stool long-lasting tenesmus, followed by relief of pains, except heavy, dull pain in back and bowels, tongue flabby, white, furred; throat dry, little thirst; < from food or drink.
Cuprum	Severe retching with the stool; cramps in abdomen, upper and lower extremities, fingers and toes; paralytic sensations in arms and feet; sweet taste in mouth with sweet stringy saliva; hard abdomen, sensitive to pressure; hiccough, comatose sleep afer vomiting; stools watery, bloody, frequent, but not very copious; urine or suppressed; exfessive thirst for cold water which relieves.

Dioscorea	Just before and during stool severe pain in sacral reguon and bowels, of a writhing drawing character; the pains radiate upward and downward, until the whole body and extremities, even the fingers and toes, become involved with spasms, eliciting shrieks from the patient; spasmodic pains in the bowels, with unusually severe tenesmus; stools like albumen, but lumpy, with straining and burning in rectum, and SENSATION AS IF THE FAECES WERE HOT; during the stool nearly fainting.
Dulcamara	Dysentery from cold damp weather; increased flow of saliva; burning itching of rectum; heat of skin; thirst, retention of urine; strangury from a cold, or from cold drinks; great straining at stool; violent cutting around navel; rectum protrudes; stools very slimy.
Erigeron	Dysentery, with burning in any part of the alimentary canal. Extreme tenesmus, with frequent small stools, streaked with blood or, bloody, and a great irritation of the urinary organs; URINATION PAINFUL OR SUPRESSED.
Ferrum Phos	Stools pure blood, blood mucus, bloody scum; yellowish, whitish, brown, with blood, like bloody fish brine, green, watery or green mucus, with blood; NO PAIN; blood dark or light; dysentery from checked perspiration in hot weather.
Gamboge	(Gummi gutt) – Chill and pain in back; bitter taste in the mouth; burning of the tongue, soreness all over; watery stools attended with colic or green mixed mucus, with burning tenesmus and prolapsus ani; offensive, frequent and copious stools, COMING OUT ALL AT ONCE, giving great relief. (Thromb., no relief)
Hamamelis	When the amount of blood in the stools is unusually large in quantitiy, amounting to an ACTUAL HEMORRHAGE; blood dark, in small clots or patches, scattered through the mucus.

Continued...

Ipecacuanha	Suitable for all dysentrties, with violent colic and tenesmus; tongue moist, yellowish or white; stools dark, almost black and fermented like frothy molasses,. Worse in the evening; tenesmus afer stool, constant nausea and vomiting.
Kali bichrom	Blackish, watery, bloody, jellylike, stringy discharges, with urgent pressure to stool, driving one out of bed in the morning; tenesmus during and after stool, TONGUE DRY, RED, SMOOTH AND CRACKED; much thirst; vomiting of bitter, sour, glairy fluids. Periodical return of DYSENTERY IN SPRING OR EARLY PART OF SUMMER. (After Canth.)
Kreosotum	Putrid stools and foetid urine, accompanied by vomiting; burning pain in bowels; palpitations with anxiety, small pulse, dry tongue; humming in ears, nosebleed etc.
Lachesis	Dark, chocolate-colored, CADAVEROUS-SMELLING STOOLS OF DECOMPOSED BLOOD, looking like charred straw; stools of mixed blood and slime, stools passed with painful straining and burning in the anus; cramping pain in the abdomen, which feels very hot; coldness; thirst, tongue red and cracked at the tip, or black and bloody.
Leptandria	Black, tarry, bilious, undigested stools, followed by great distress in the liver; mushy with weak feeling in bowels, of mixed mucus, flocculent and watery, with yellow bile and blood; stools of pure blood; pain bowels after stool, but no tenesmus, < morning, as soon as he moves.
Lilium	Bloody mucous stools every half hour; constant urging to stool and much backache; after stool a feeling as if more would pass, < from slightest motion, constant thirst for water; frequent desire to urinate; tenderness over left ovary; prolapsus uteri.
Lycopodium	Chronic dysentery; stools shaggy, of reddish mucus, putrid; much flatulence; constant and distressing pressure in rectum; urgent straining, with shuddering and sense of insufficient evacuation.

DYSENTERY REMEDIES	
Magnesia Carb	Bloody mucus mixed with the green watery stool, sinking to the brown stools, with blood, like bloody fish brine; green; watery or green mucus, with blood dark light; dysentery from checked perspiration in hot water.
Magnesia Phos	Terrible pains in rectum witgh every stool, as if from a prolonged spasm of the muscles employed in defaecation, muicturatio, or in both.
Mercurius	Excoriating discharges; cutting in the lower part of the abdomen, at night, the abdomen is externally cold to the touch; cutting stich in lower abdomen, from right to left, and aggravated by walking; faecal putrid taste in the mouth; nausea, with vertigo, obscured vision, and flashes of heat; offensive persipation; the pains are increased BEFORE the stool and DURING the stool, with violent tenesmus; the PAINS ARE RATHER INCREASED AFTER A STOOL, and sometimes they extend to the back; during the stool hot sweat on the forehead, which soon becomes cold and sticky; frequent discharge of pure blood or bloody green mucus, like stirred eggs, screams during stool (in children). Aggravation during night till about 3 A.M
Muriatic. acid	Dysenteric stools, BLOOD AND SLIME SEPARATED. As soon as he begins to move strong urging compels haste, stools profuse, dark-brown, gelatinous; pressing, drawing tired pain in lumbar region, prostration and drowsiness, wants to lie down all day
Merc.cor	Almost constant cutting pains in abdomen and intolerable, almost ineffectual pressing, straining and tenesmus; only frequent scanty discharges of bloody slime, day and night; SEVERE PAINS IN RECTUM, CONTINUE AFTER STOOL, with pressing downword in front of abdomen below the navel (Opunt.); faintness, weakness and shudering, limbs feel bruised and trembling; cold face and hands, with small and feeble pulse; < in fall, hot days and cool nights, afer midnight; burning and tenesmus conjoinatly of rectum and bladder; suppression of secretion or retention of urine

Continued...

Nitric acid	DIPHTHERITIC DYSENTERY; burning in rectum towards perineum, with ineffectual urging; straining without stool; stools bloody, with tenesmus; dryness of throat; violent thirst; intermittent pulse; anxiety and general uneasiness, exhaustion
Nux Vomica	Stools, small, slimy, bloody, with urging, TENESMUS CEASING AFTER STOOL; like pitch with blood; pressing pains in loins and upper part of sacral region, with sensation as if broken; longing for brandy; milk sours on stomach; great debility with oversensitiveness of all the senses; hypochondriac mood.
Opuntia vulg	Excoriating sick feeling in LOWER PART OF ABDOMEN; with sensation as if all the bowels settled down in lower part of abdomen; bowels move oftener than natural with urgent desire for stool.
Petroleum	Dysesntric diarrhoea, consisting of bloody mucus, followed by much pressing; as if all large quantities were yet to be expelled; weak and dizzy after stool; < mornings from urgent desire for stool (Teste).
Phosphorus	PAINLESS discharges of blood and mucus, the anus remaining open; desire for stools as often as she turns on her left side (Arn.).
Plumbum	Burning in anus during stool and long-lasting, severe tenesmus afterwards; frequent and almost fruitless efforts to stool, which is bloody, watery, offensive; cutting pains with violent screaming, anus feels as if drawn upward; retraction of abdomen.
Podophyllum	Severe straining during stool, with emission of much flatulence, mucous stools, with spots and streaks of blood, great thirst, but no appetite, stools yellow, green, brownish, watery, mucus streaked with blood, with heat in rectum, flashes of heat running up the back, painful tenesmus and decent of rectum; great sensation of weakness in rectum.

Pulsitilla	Discharges white, slimy, whitish-coated tongue; pappy, sticky taste, without thirst, great difficulty in breathing; all worse at night; dystenteric stools of clear yellow, red or green slime; pain in back, straining; tenesmus from anus up along sacarum; dysentery during cholera times; discharge of blood and mucus during stool; face pallid; fainting; dysuria; frequent stools of mucus only after dysentery.
Rhododendron	Dysentery in summer, during thunderstorm; stool tardy, papascent, requiring much urging.
Rhus tox	Stools watery, mucous and bloody, with nausea, tearing down the thighs and much tenesmus; like the washings of meat; tenesmus vesicae; jeklly like discharges; tenesmus and urging before stool, with remission after stool; changes position often to get relief from tearing pains down thighs, < at night, after getting wet.
Staphisgria	Cutting pain before and after stool; tenesmus in rectumand bladder during stool, <after eating, and drinking cold water.
Sulphur	Dysentric stools at night, with colic and violent tenesmus; blood in mucus in thready streaks; frequent unsuccessful desire for stool; WITH THE STOOL TENESMUS CEASES. BUT MUCUS AND BLOOD ARE STILL BEING DISCHARGED; prolapsu ani at night; cutting pains while urging at stool, > by dry heat; chills on lower part of body and lassitude
Thrombidium	Abdominal pains begin while eating, are not relieved by stools, which are unceasing, occurring every half-hour, accompanied by tenesmus; flatus give no relief; brown fluid stools, with or without bloody streaks; discharge of mucus, soft faeces or pus, or blood and mucus with violent colic, causing the patient to scream; prolapsus ani, skin dry, tongue coated, thirst moderate.
Zincum (Zinc,sulph)	Chrinic dysentery; stools frequent, mall, pitch-like or thin, with pale blood; involuntary; ext reme emaciation; great desire for food, which fails to be assimilated; twitching of muscles, jerking of muscles during sleep.

Continued...

JUANDIS REMEDIES	
Chionanathus	Catararhal jaundice with rumbling; jaundice returning every summer, soreness and griping. Tongue and eyes yellow. Urine contains traces of bile and sugar. Jaundice with suppression of menses. Constipation with clay colour stool.
Chammomila	Jaundice caused by a fit of anger or by any undue excitement. Congestion of liver, loss of appetite, nausea, foul and slimy taste in mouth, pinching and twisting pains in the abdomen.
Chelidonium	This should follow Sulphur after one day. It is specific for jaundice and is normally given in 6th dilution. Yellowness of the conjunctiva; sallow complexion; bitter taste, deep red colour of tongue; tenderness of liver on pressure; brown-red urine and light clay coloured stools.
Hydrastis	Catarrhal jaundice with sharp stitching pains and excessive secretions of tenacious mucus. Nausea and vomiting. Atrophy of the liver. Tongue swollen showing marks of teeth with white or yellow coating.
Myrica Cerifera	An important remedy for catarrhal jaundice. There is dull headache – worse in the morning, the eyes have a dingy, dirty, yellow hue, tongue is coated yellow. Patient is weak and complains of muscular soreness and aching in the limbs with slow pulse and dark urine. Pain in the right side below the ribs. No appetite – desire for acids – un-refreshing sleep.
Merc. Sol	A leading remedy for jaundice; accelerated pulse, yellowish tinge of the conjunctiva; slightly coated tongue; constipated; pale and dry consistence of feacus of deep yellow colour. Profuse sweat with relief. Increased secretions, especially saliva; flabby tongue; metallic taste. Sensitiveness over the region of liver which is swollen and hard with stinging and stitching pains.
Nux Vomica	With tendency to piles and constipation. Foul, musty or bitter taste. Aversion to food. Throbbing pain in the region of liver. Fainting fits.

Ptelia T	Jaundice with hyperaemia of liver. Griping in stomach with dry mouth
Sulphur 200	Always start treatment of jaundice with this remedy. It should also be thought of for completing the cure

Or Use Hepatica to normalize the liver – 3 times in a day one hour before meals for about one month after the jaundice symptoms are completely eliminated

DIET: Cane-sugar juice, or glucose very often – No fats to be allowed – Plenty of fruits and easily digestable food, fat removed butter milk – coconut water – Broken milk to be squeezed in a cloth and the liquid thereof be given during cute stage

Juandis (Malignant) Remedies	
Ars. Alb	In last stages of malignant jaundice. There may be fever with restlessness and thirst for small quantities of water at short intervals.
Lachesis	Indicated in persons who are anaemic, nervous and sensitive. They are worse after sleep, after hot drinks and in a worm room. Urine foamy, dark and almost black. Burning and itching of the whole body. Blueness along entire course of veins.
Phosphorous	Indicated only in the early stage of malignancy of the disease. Enlargement and induration of liver. Acute atrophy of the liver. Interstitial hepatitis. Malignant jaundice.

After the jaundice symptoms are completely eliminated:

Cardus Mar Q (mother tincture) 3 to 6 drops @ 8 am., and 8 pm. For about 20 days

Or Use Hepatica to normalize the liver – 3 times in a day one hour before meals for about one month after the jaundice symptoms are completely eliminated

DIET: Cane-sugar juice, or glucose very often – No fats to be allowed – Plenty of fruits and easily digestable food, fat removed butter milk – coconut water – Broken milk to be squeezed in a cloth and the liquid thereof be given during cute stage

Continued...

SPLEEN REMEDIES (Remedies)	
Aranea Diadema	Enlargement of spleen due to chronic effects of malaria, Languor, lassitude and constant chilliness are useful symptoms
Bryonia	For simple congestion and inflammation of spleen with stitching and tearing pains which are worse from motion and better by rest.
Ceanothus	The head remedy and inflammation of spleen. It is normally used in mother tincture(Q) in drop doses. Deep seated pains in the splenic region, deep stitches, worse in damp weather. Chills and fever, floating and displaced spleen.
China	The next best remedy for enlargement of spleen when there is congestion, swelling and stitching in the spleen due to protracted and severe fevers.
Capscicum	Useful for sensitive, swollen and enlarged spleen.
Succinum Acid	For improving the condition and function of the spleen

GASTRO-INTESTINAL TOXEMIA

Synonyms: Intestinal intoxication, systemic intoxication.

Aetiology: Constipation is a frequent predisposing cause of both the acute and chronic forms. Excess of food which may be indigestible **or** has already undergone fermentation is also an active cause. A lack of fresh air and exercise and inividaual peculiarities are also casual factors. Toxic agents developed within the body, the result of defective elimination **or** faulty cell metabolism, are prominent in the **Aetiology.**

Pathology:

While the contents of the intestinal tract are naturally toxic, yet this toxicity is increased by bacterial fermentation of food while albumen and neclein may produce profound systemic toxemia. The changes in these two substances are the result of the action of enzymes or bacteria. The poisons produced by the bacteria in the intestinal tract may be derived from three sources. The components of dead bacteria may furnish proteins, some of which are poisonous, living bacteria in the intestinal canal may excrete ferments which produce nervous symptoms and intestinal toxemia; still another source is found to be substances produced by the bacteria from the culture media, such as the *ptomaines,* the virulence of which depends upon the micro-organisms which produce them and the food material upon which they have been cultivated. Other substances that may produce this condition are indol, skatol etc., dilatation of the stomach and drooping of the viscera comprising the gastro-intestinal canal may be responsible for it. Owing to the great irritability and immaturity of the nervous system in children, intestinal toxemia is responsible for many of the disturbances that affect infants and children. A small amount of poisonous material will produce fever and convulsions. This condition is responsible for many of the ills of certain children. Chronic intestinal toxaemia is produced by the same poisons by the same poisons that produce the acute form, but it is absorbed in similar quantities and over a much longer period of time.

Symptoms:

The patient is usually anaemic and malnutrition is apparent. Headaches of a toxic character are complained of, as well as malaise, mental depression, restlessness at night, incontinence of urine, buzzing in the ears, disturbance of the sight and vertigo. The reflexes are exaggerated, nervous symptoms as hyperesthesia, psychoses, convulsive disturbances are present. The urine contains an excess of *indican, calcium oxalate, uric acid and ethereal sulphates.* Meterorism and tympanites are present and there are eructations which are preceded by a burning sensation in the stomach, in the esophagus and pharynx. In nearly all these cases pyorrhoea alveolaris present. Acid vomiting may occur. *The acidity is more frequently dependent upon acetic acid than upon hydroclhoric acid.* On account of the acidity of the intestinal contents, irritating of the mucous membrane, diarrhoea results or constipation and diarrhea may alternate. Examination of the colon will show it to be distended with feacal material.

GASTRO-INTESTINAL TOXEMIA – Remedies	
Acid Carbolic	The bowels area inactive, or there is an alternate diarrhea and constipation, and there are emissions of putrid flatus and the stools are extremely fetid. The breath is offensive. Patient complains much of the time of dull frontal headache and of a sensation of a band about the head. The tongue is coated, there are constant eructations and rumbling of gas in the abdomen. Palpitation reveals a tenderness over the colon. Complains of various nervous sensations and a profound prostration, while at times the surface of the body is covered with a cold perspiration.
Baptisia	Is frequently indicated in cases in which there are evidences of a septic condition of the intestinal tract. The patient complains of stupefying headache, with confusion of ideas. The complaint of great weakness and a sensation of soreness over the body. The breath and, intestinal gas is offensive, patient recognizes that when the flatus is not passed readily, he becomes weak and exhausted, as if poisoned.
Hydrastis	This remedy should be studied in those cases in which there is evidence of an atonic condition and deficient assimilation of food, and as a result the patient is anemic and complains of fatigue. The natural secretions of the mucous surfaces are increased and are abnormal both in quantity and quality. At first they are clear, white, transparent and presents a slimy appearance. There is a dull aching pain referred to the region of the stomach, a sensation of weakness and emptiness. The bowels are constipated and there is usually a history of cathartics having been employed

Iris Vers	Should be studied in cases in which the patient complains of a dull heavy headache. It begins with a blur before the eyes and it may be conveyed to the forehead, or it may extend to one or both of the temples, but usually the right. Occasionally it is throbbing or hammering in character. It is atended with nausea at times, vomiting of sour, bilious material. Patient complains of a putrid taste. There are rumbling and indications of large quantities of gas in the intestines and complaints of great debility.
Psorinum	Should be studied in those case in which the well-selected remedy does not afford the desired relief, or when they have not fully recovered from an acute disease. The patient is continaually chilly. There are foul odors from the body.

ENTERALGIA

Synonym: Intestinal colic.

Aetiology: This is observed especially in anemic, hysteric, neurasthenic patients when subjected to severe mental strain, anxiety, and violent emotions. Tabetic patients are subject to attacks of severe intestinal pain known as "intestinal crises". Toxic influences that result from lead and copper produce severe intestinal pain, as do gout, intestinal worms, feacal accumulations, gaseous accumulations and indulgence in certain kinds of foods. Reflex intestinal pains may have their origin in diseases of the uterus, kidneys and liver, while peritonitic adhesions occasionally excite attacks.

Symptoms:

The principal symptom is abdominal pain which is usually referred to the umbilical region and may radiate from this for a considerable distance. It may change locations. The pain varies in severity from a slight abdominal griping, cutting. stabbing, pinching or burning pain to one of such intensity that the patient writhes, while the skin becomes pale and cool, cold sweat appears and the face presents an expression of fear. The pulse is small, hard and the heart sounds are faint. Syncope and general clonic and contraction of the *cremasteric* muscles. The frequency of the recurrence and the duration of an attack is always problematic. It may terminate suddenly following vomiting or the escape of gasses from the intestines. The abdominal walls may be rigid, tympanitic or relaxed. Firm pressure usually mitigates the pain.

ENTERALGIA: – Remedies	
Ars. alb.	Indicated in those who are anxious, fearful, restless, full of anguish. In whom the attacks come on suddenly after eating and drinking, especially after partaking of ice water, cake or ice cream; periodical attacks due to malarial influence; neuralgic attacks followed by great restlessness and intolerable suffering; paroxysm attended by nausea and a vomiting, or with thin, watery stools; pains worse at night, also after eating and drinking, better from warm applications.
Alumina	Should be remembered in spare, dry thin subjects who complain of paroxysmal pains, with dysponea, worse when stooping, violent cutting pains, principally in the evening, succeeded by oppression of the chest, colic-like pain, followed by diarrhoea and pain in the region of the kidneys, pinching and lacerating pain, with chilliness in the abdomen, relieved by heat.
Belladonna	Is indicated in bilious, lymphatic, plethoric persons who complain of violent cutting, clutching, clawing pains in various parts of abdomen, constantly shifting about, appearing and disappearing suddenly; light pressure aggravates, but hard pressure relieves. Thirsty, but drinks little, as drinking aggravates the pains; tendency to cerebral hyperaemia; worse until evening and after midnight.

ENTERALGIA: – Remedies	
Colocynth	When this remedy is indicated the pains appear to radiate from the umbilicus, are of a sharp, cutting, darting or twisting character, and occur in paroxysm; relieved by bending double or by hard pressure; coffee and smoking relieve, but food and other drinks usually aggravate.
Chammomilla	Is indicated in those of a nervous, irritable, excitable temperament, who are over sensitive to pain and complain of colic like pains in the region of the navel, also lower down on both sides, with pain in the hollow of the back as if broken; abdomen swollen and drum-like; flatus passed in small quantities without relief; relieved by warm applications.
Cuprum Met	Indicated in those who complain of mental and physical exhaustion from over exertion of the mind and loss of sleep. They complain of violent cutting, drawing, intermittent pains. Abdomen retracted and sore to touch; pains cause the patient to utter fearful screams; very restless and uneasy, constantly tossing about; worse by drinking cold water.
Cuprum Ars	This remedy should be carefully studied and compared with the former remedy.
Magnesia Phos	Indicated in dark complexioned, thin, nervous persons who complain of sharp, cutting, stabbing, itching, lightning like pains, relieved by pressure and hot applications.
Opium	Indicated in those with light hair, lax muscles and want of bodily irritability. They complain of colic, violent cutting pains in the abdomen, as if made with a knife; constipation, with hard and distended abdomen; pains worse before and after stool; hypochondriac regions painful when touched.
Plumbum	Is indicated when the disease is of the spinal region and there is a rapid and excessive emaciation. Complaints of excruciating pains in the umbilical region, shooting to other parts, and moderated by pressure. Recti muscles hard and knotty; abdomen retracted to the utmost extent; ameliorated by hard pressure and by friction; obstinate constipation, pains resembling lead colic, but due to some other cause.

Continued...

| Podophyllum | Should be studied in the case of those with a bilious temperament who suffer from gastro intestinal derangements and lead colic; frequently recurring attacks accompanied by retraction of the abdominal walls; severe straining during stool with escape of flatus; morning aggravatioins; attacks renewed by eating and drinking. |

APPENDICITIS

Definition:

This is an infection of the vermiform appendix which may be either catarrhal, chronic or recurrent; and which may terminate either in recovery, suppuration, gangrene and perforation or abscess formation. The caput colic is frequently involved, giving rise to typhilits and peri-typhilitis.

Aetiology:

This is dependent upon injury or infective agent, or both. The injury may be the result of a feacal concretion, or in rare cases a fruit stone, or other foreign bodies within the appendix, in other cases a virulent type of bacteria is operative, as the *bacillus coli communis, the proteus vulgaris, the streptococcus, the typhoid bacillus or actinomycossis.*

If the predisposing causes, stricture of the proximal portion of the appendix (Gerlach'valve) should be mentioned, as this interferes with the proper drainage of the appendix. The blood supply may be so interfered with as to favour infection or the position of appendix may be such as to favour it.

Pathology:

It should be remembered that the appendix is a glandular organ presenting certain points similar to the tonsils, and like them is subject to *follicular, mucous, submucus, infective, exudative* and *ulcerative disorders.* Preceding the catarrhal form there is usually a history of constipation and indiscretion of diet. After passing through the inflammatory stages this form subsides but there remains an increased vascularity of the appendix that renders it susceptible to recurrent attacks. Obliterating appendicitis is but the later stage of the catarrhal form in which the ulceration is produced by feacal concretion of a foreign body within the appendix gradually passes to perforation. This is usually near the apex. The concretion passes through the wall of the appendix into the abdominal cavity with the septic discharge and causes septic *peritonitis or a perityphlitic* abcess. If there has been adhesion of the appendix and the peritoneum, both are perforated, and the abcess becomes extra-peritoneal. Adhesions are common in all directions, while pleurisy is at times met with. In some cases concretions are found obliterating the canal; in other cases there is ulceration of the interior of the appendix; while in others there is an obliterating appendicitis. In the gangrenous type, rapid sloughing of a part or the whole of the wall of the organ takes place. The condition is a grave one and may result in a general peritonitis of the severest type.

The attending inflammatory process varies from a simple peri-appendicular exudates, which forms adhesions with surrounding organs, to one of a much severer form, which occupies the right iliac fossa. The quality of pus in the cavity varies from a drachma to a pint or over. It may break through its adhesions and discharge into the peritoneal cavity, towards the intestines, bladder or vagina. It may rupture through the abdominal wall. There may be metastatic abscess of the liver.

Symptoms:

The attack is usually ushered in by a sudden intense pain in the right iliac fossa. This is frequently localized at a point midway between the anterior superior spine of the ileum and the umbilicus (McBrney's point). The pain may radiate from this towards the umbilicus, epigastrium, the groin and the testicle. It is attended with periods of excerbation. An absence of pain is no indication that the disease is not present and not progressing. In the majority of cases nausea and vomiting are present. The pulse is usually rapid, while the temperature may reach 104 F although the temperature gives but little information regarding the severity of the case. Constipation is usually present during the early stages, but little information regarding the severity of the case. Constipation is usually present during the early stages, but diarrhea and constipation may alternate. There is rigidity of the right abdominal muscles or there may be circumscribed rigidity over the region of the appendix. But in these cases a tumour may be felt at the lower border of the ileum. In some cases, and especially in children, the disease may come on insidiously pain and fever be totally absent. There may be some colicky pain in this region. If the case is one of milk catarrhal appendicitis the symptoms are slight, and often hardly noticeable; they continue for two to three days, when the patient gradually recovers. But when upon or about the third day after the onset of the symptoms, a localized superficial oedema appears, when a doughy mass is felt at the seat of pain which gradually assumes shape to the touch, it is likely that suppuration has taken place and a white blood count will show a leucocytosis of from 20000 to 30000 and perforation imminent.

If adhesions have had time to form, the tumour may remain after perforation has taken place, but if perforatioin has taken place early before the adhesions have formed there is usually a chill, vomiting, shock, a more or less diffused pain, a quickened pulse and an increased temperature. The tumour is not felt and the symptoms are those a diffused peritonitis. The patient usually lies upon his back with right thigh flexed on the pelvis.

APPENDICITIS: Remedies	
Ars.Alb.	Is indicated when the patient is greatly prostrated, restless with a sensation of burning. All conditions are worse during the night and from cold and are better from heat. There is a constant desire for a mouthful of water, but the patient vomits immediately after eating or drinking

Belladonna	This remedy should be studied when the attack and the pain appear suddenly. The parts are extremely sensitive to the touch or motion, even of the bed. The pulse is rapid and there are all the indications of intense congestion and approaching inflammation.
Bryonia Alb	May be studied when there are indications of peritonitis. There is pain, soreness and sensitiveness in the ilio – caecal region. The pain is aggravated upon the slightest attempt to move. Patient is thirsty and wishes to drink large quantities of water. The lips, tongue and throat are dry. The bowels are constipated.
Cantharis	Is indicated when there are sharp, stitching burning pains. The patient is restless with a pale, death-like face. There is violent urinary tenesmus and strangury, and the stools are apt to consist of reddish mucus like scraping of the intestines.
Calcarea Sulph	Should be studied where suppuration is present and the patient is cachectic, the face is pale yellow, pinched, old looking and there is a picture of weakness, has lost his nerve, is weak and faint hearted.
Hepar Sulf	Is useful in suppurative cases where thorough drainage has been established. The patient gives a history of repeated suppuration upon the slightest provocation. He is extremely sensitive to drafts of air, takes cold easily, and is oversensitive to pain.
Merc. Corr	Is useful in those cases when there is present a hard, painful, indurated mass with alternate chills and heat. The face is pale, tongue is broad and flabby with white coating. The bowels may be constipated or the evacuations be slimy.
Lachesis	Should be remembered in the typhoid septic cases. The parts are dark coloured and the patient is worse after sleep.
Rhus Tox	Given in cases that assume a typhoid type. The abdomen is distended and painful, the patient is in such distress that he must move and finds but a momentary relief. The parts are red, swollen and sensitive.

Continued...

| Silicea | Is indicated in much the same conditions as Hepar Sulf, suppuration is present and the drainage is taking place. The patient is cachectic, the face is pale yellow, pinched, old looking and there is a picture of weakness, has "lost his nerve" is weak and fain hearted. |

ACCUMULATION OF GAS IN THE INTESTINES

Synonyms: Meterosim, tympanies, flatulence

Meteorism and tympanites are terms used to describe abnormal accumulations of gas in the intestines. The term flatulence is used to indicate a great formation of gases that are removed by eructations or by belching. Physiologically the intestines contain a certain amount of gas. Carbon dioxide in the intestines is partially derived by diffusion from the blood-vessels in the intestines. Hydrogen, ammonia, methane and sulphuretted hydrogen are wolly derived from fermentation and putrefaction of the intestinal tract.

Aetiology:

Aerophagy or air swallowing is noticed in hysterical women. Constipation is present in many cases and assists fermentation. Large quantities of fermentable substances in the intestines with bacteria and fungi favour the development of gases. Meterorism may be dependent upon intestinal obstruction, and in diffused peritonitis due to arrested muscular action of the intestines.

There is a form of meteorism noticed in hysterical subjects (tympanites hystericas) which in some cases gives rise to a diffused distension of the abdomen; while in other cases it is circumscribed (phantom tumour). The particular etiological factor in these cases is not determined

Symptoms:

There is a symmetrical development of the abdomen, although it may be localized. Percussion gives a meteroistic note, owing to the diaphragm being forced up, the pulmonary percussion note is dull, the apex of the heart is displaced. Respirations become shallow, rapid and costal in character. The patient becomes cyanotic. The jugular veins are distended. The patient may complain of great pain. In some cases the condition is localised and phantom tumour is present.

ACCUMULATION OF GAS IN THE INTESTINES – Remedies	
Arg.Nit.	Should be remembered in neurotic subjects, when the eructation is annoying and the gas escapes with much noise.
Gratiola	Should be remembered in cases in which there is great distension of the abdomen and of the stomach, with lassitude and constriction of the throat & rectum, and with constipation.
Lycopodium	Is of service when the colon is distended and the bowels are constipated
Lobelia	When there is the sensation of a lump in the throat which interferes with respiration and deglution.
Nux Mosch.	Has great distension after eating

WORMS: Tape-worm (Cestodes)

Varieties:

Tenia Saginata or beef tape-worm, tenia solium or pork tape-worm, both ricephalus or tenia latus, the fish tape-worm.

Symptoms:

These may attain considerable size, and may infest the host for a long period without giving rise to any symptoms. The positive diagnosis can be made only by finding segments of the worm in the stool. There may be colicky pains in the abdomen, and alternate diarrhea and constipation; at times there is nausea, especially when the stomach is empty. Anemia is common, especially if the *bothriocephalus latus* is the parasite present. In some cases vertigo, chorea and epilepsy are present. All the symptoms are aggravated when the stomach is empty.

WORMS: Tape-worm – Cestodes – Remedies	
Cucurbita pepo semen(Pumpkin seed)	From one to three ounces of the pulp of the seed macerated and mixed with honey and spread like jam on thin slice of bread, is mild and highly useful.
Flixmas (male ferm)	Is employed extensively. The dose is from one to two drachms, preferably in capsules. If there is a tendency to vomit after taking it, this may be controlled by swallowing black coffee or lemonade. A saline should be employed before and following its use rather than castor oil as the latter cause the toxic principle, filicic acid, to be absorbed.
Kamala	One-half ounce to be taken in two doses diluted with water
Kousso	An infusion with flowers, one ounce to eight ounces of water. This should be taken in the morning and followed by a catharitic.
Pelletierine tannate	Is used by many. It is administered in capsule, preceded and followed by a cathartic. The dose for an adult is four grains. It should be given with great care to children.
Homoeo remedies Napthalinum, Thymol, Santonin and Carbolic Acid also to be studied	

ASCARIS LUMBRICOIDES

The symptoms they give rise to are never so distinctive that the cause may be definitely determined. There is abdominal pain, borborygmus; irregularity of the bowel movement, itching of the anus, anorexia, nausea, vomiting offensive breath: while reflexly they may produce vertigo, headache, inequality of the pupils, eclampsia, chorea, and muscular spasms. The patient often complains of itching of the nose, and digs the fingers into the nostrils. He often is emaciated, pallid and has dark rings about the eyes. The worms may occupy the whole lumen of the bowel and give rise to intestinal obstruction. They wander about and may close the ductus choledoctus or pass through the stomach, esophagus, and have been known to pass during sleep into the larynx and be the cause of death. They have been found in intestinal perforation, appendiceal and perineal abcesses.

Ascaris Lumbricoides – (Remedies)	
Cina	Is of service in children when the pupils are dilated, the face is pale and there are dark rings about the eyes. The child grinds its teeth during sleep, picks and bores at its nose, and cries out during sleep.
Mercurius	Has been of service when the general symptoms call for it.
Naphthalin	Has been employed and should be studied
Santonin	Is indicted in many cases when the presence of the worm has been demonstrated. The symptoms are similar to those of cina
Also study Ant,Crud., Stannum and Spigelia	

ACUTE PERITONITIS

Definition: This is an acute inflammation of the peritoneum.

Aetiology: It is the result of wounds, bruises, and perforation of the stomach, duodenum, and small intestines, of the appendix, and the colon in malignant diseases. It results from rupture of hydrated cysts and of abscess of the various organs. The pathogenic germs that give rise to peritonitis are *bacilli coli communis, streptococci, staphyloccoci, pneumonococci and tubercule bacilli.*

Pathology: In the early stages the peritoneum is roughened and congested. The intestines are distended with gas. In a short time there is an inflammatory exudates on the surface of the peritoneum. This may consist of fibrin only, or serum and fibrin, pus or bloody serum, especially peritoneum. This may consist of fibrin only, or serum and fibrin, or pus or bloody serum, especially if due to an external wound. The coils of intestine are more or less adherent to one another. In cases of perforation, carcinoma and rupture of the uterus, the serum is mixed with septic material and the odor is foul. The amount of fluid varies.

In long standing cases the adhesions become dense bands of tissue. In the circumscribed form the adhesions may wall off collections of pus or fluid.

Symptoms: There is an acute abdominal pain with tympanites, nausea, vomiting, constipation and elevation of temperature. The pulse is small, rapid and tense. The face is drawn and the expression is anxious, the breathing is shallow, rapid and of the thoracic type. The abdominal pain and tenderness are so intense that the patient dreads the slightest movement or pressure. The thighs are flexed on the abdomen to relax the abdominal parieties. The body is often covered with a cold sweat and collapse may be present. Should pus form, there will be rigors and hectic fever. If the process is putrid, death speedily results from septic intoxication.

Treatment: The patient should be kept quiet in bed. All pressure should be removed from the abdomen. The diet should consist of nothing but fluids. External applications, either in the form of a poultice or ice bag, should be used, according as the patient prefers. Heat may be applied in the form of a hot water bag, or a flaunel wrung out of hot water and covered with oil silk, or by a flax seed poultice, changed often and kept hot by means of oil silk.

ACUTE PERITONITIS: Remedies	
Aconite	This remedy should be studied in the early history of those cases in which the attack is the result of exposure and cold. The skin is dry and hot, the pulse is full, hard and rapid, the respirations are rapid and the temperture is high. The patient is anxious and restless; there is great thirst with vomiting. The urine is scanty and of a dark red colour. The abdomen is swollen burning and hot. There are sharp cutting pains through the abdomen.

Ars. Alb.	Should be carefully compared with Veratrum Album. The pains are violent and colicky. There is the sensation of burning and thirst and the general symptoms that should lead to its selection
Belladonna	When this remedy is indicated the pulse is full and strong. There is much throbbing of the carotids. The face is flushed, the eye seems to protrude and the pupils are dilated. The abdomen is distended, painful and the patient complains of burning, cutting colicky pains which are worse from the slightest motion, or pressure. When this remedy fails to give the desired result, **Atropine** should be compared
Bryonia	Should be studied when serous effusion has taken place. There are stitching, lancinating pains in the bowels which are rendered worse on motion. The patient is thirsty and desires large quantities of water. The mouth, lips and tongue are very dry. The tongue has a white coating. The bowels are constipated and the patient complains of nausea when compelled to move.
Cantharis	Is indicated in cases that are attended with violent burning and cutting pains in the abdomen and extensive tympanites. There is great prostration and painful urination
Colocynthis	Is indicted in cases characterized by stinging, lancinating, burning pains in the abdomen which distended and tympanitic. The patient complains of violent, distressing pains during stool. The pulse is small and rapid. The extremities are cold. Enteritis may be associated with peritonitis
Sulphur	Fills a place and is indicated in these cases when another remedy, although indicated, has not caused absorption of the fluid. In these cases there is a lack of reaction, recovery is not taking place, and the patient complains of great weakness. If a hectic fever is present, or if ulceration is taking place, the use of this remedy is but a loss of time.

If suppuration takes place and drainage is established, Silicea, Hepar Sulph and Calcarea Sulph should be studied.

Continued...

When a typhoid condition develops, Arnica, Baptisia, Muriatic Acid and Rhus tox should be studied,
When suppuration is threatened, Chin Ars., Mer Corr., and Sulphur should be studied.

ASCITES

Synonym: Hydroperitoneum

Etiology: This occurs either as a result of an increased blood pressure in the branches of portal veins or abnormal permeability of the walls of the veins. There may be a portal stasis the result of chronic interstitial hepatitis or other diseases of the liver. Stenosis of the hepatic veins is result of a chronic interstitial hepatitis or other diseases of the liver. Stenosis of the hepatic veins is an occasional cause, as are nephritis, carcinoma, pulmonary tuberculosis, chronic diarrhea and chronic suppuration. Chylous ascites is caused either by an obstruction of the thoracic duct or lacteals.

ASCITES: Remedies	
Apocynum	Useful in many of these cases. It should be given in doses of twenty to thirty drops of an infusion **or** from five to eight drops of tincture four times a day. Some patients do not take this remedy well.
Ars. Alb.	Should be studied in those with cirrhotic liver, and who are alcoholics, and in the aged who suffer from weak heart.
Cinchona	Should be remembered in those who suffer from anemia following diarrhea
Digitialis	Should be thought of especially if the heart is dilated and a general anascara is present
Aurum Mur Natrum, Plumbum Acetate should be studied in cases of hepatic cirrhosis	
Helleborus, Iodine and Iodoform should be remembered in those cases in which the ascites is dependent upon tuberculosis **Bryonia and Terebinthina** are also indicated at times	

HERNIA

When a part of an organ protrudes through an abdominal opening or in an abnormal way, called a Hernia. A groin (inguinal) hernia occurs when part of the intestine bulges through a weak spot in the abdominal wall at inguinal canal, **Cases of Inguinal hernia come across often for treatment** than **other** category. **The other category of Hernias are** Umblical, Incarcerated, or Strangulated inguinal hernia, Femoral hernia.

In all these cases the related screen reports are to be examined carefully. Each case should be examined very deeply, and Aetiology (i.e. route cause) thereof and accordingly the selection of remedy to be decided.

Inguinal Hernia – Remedies	
Allium Cepa	Pressure in left Inguinal ring hernia left groin most protruded and strangulated, restlessness and fever.
Coffea	Strangulated inguinal hernia, taxis becomes easier after a cup of strong coffee.
Lycopodium	Right Inguinal region, full distended abdomen, with cold feet, grumbling and gurgling in abdomen; spasmodic contraction in abdomen; lacerating stitches in hernia; right inguinal hernia from relaxation produced by the chewing of tobacco.
Psorinum	Inguinal Hernia; pain through right groin when walking; abdomen distended.
Silica	Inguinal Hernia; the child is very tender to the touch around the tumor.
Aconite	Violent inflammation of the incarcerated hernia, with burning pains in abdomen as from hot coals, extreme sensitiveness to contact; bitter bilious vomiting; anguish and cold sweat.
Aurum Met	Pressure in abdominal ring as if hernia would protrude while sitting; protrusion of inguinal hernia, with great cramp like pains; INGUINAL HERNIA OF CHILDREN, umbilical hernia of children, caused by crying.

Continued...

Belladona	Constriction of abdomen around the navel, as if a lump or a ball would form there; feeling as if a hard body pressed from within outward at right inguinal ring, the part of feeling hard to touch while sitting with the body bent forward; distension of abdomen, neither hard nor painful; colic as if a spot in abdomen were seized by nails; intense local inflammation.
Borax	**Infantile hernia**; the child dreads a downward motion; is frightened by every little noise; does not thrive; brown, watery diarrhoea.
Bryonia	Hard swelling of hypochondria and around navel; painful twisting around umbilicus, with stitches; constipation.
Calc. Carb.	**Infantile hernia**; considerable distension of abdomen, with colic; constant gurgling in abdomen; very open fontanelles, perspires about head when sleeping.
Hernia of other category – Remedies	
Carbo Veg	Great anxiety, with uneasiness in abdomen; meteorism, with loud rumbling, foetid or odourless flatus; clothing oppresses, can hardly be endured; abdomen feels as if hanging heavily; walks bent; foulness of parts as if strangulated.
Cubeba	Femoral hernia; sensation of weight, pressure and pain about femoral ring; downword pressure and weight, < after walking, riding, lifting and especially before and during menses.
Nitric Acid	**Inguinal hernia, also of children also of children**; drawing pain in abdomen, with shuddering; frequent pinching and rumbling in abdomen, which is excessively sensitive.
Nux Vom.	Strangulated, bruised pain in bowels, as if they were raw and sore, **frequent protrusion of inguinal hernia**, with red or yellowish foci; some tenderness from pressure on the tumour; nausea, vomiting, constipation; sensation of weakness in abdominal ring; left side mostly affected (Lyc: right side)
Nux Mosch	Umblical hernia; abdomen enormously distended, cutting pinching about navel > from pressure; sore navel; even ulcerated.

Sulphuric Acid	Colic, with sensation as if a hernia would protrude; violent protrusion of an inguinal hernia; sour vomit, first water, then food; vomiting of drunkards; sensation of trembling, without visible trembling.
Tabacum	Strangulated hernia, pallor of face, extremities cold and covered with clammy sweat; nausea, accompanied by burning heat in abdomen, rest of body cold; patient persists in uncovering abdomen.
Verat alb.	INCARCERATED HERNIA, not inflamed, antiperistaltic action, hiccough, cold sweat, nausea with sensateiun of fainting and violent thirst: INTUSSUSCEPTION OF BOWELS, great anguish, rushes about bent double, pressing the abdomen; cold feeling in abdomen, great sinking of strength, and empty feeling.

ASCARIS LUMBRICOIDES

Symptoms:

The symptoms they give rise to are never so distinctive that the cause may be definitely determined. There is abdominal pain, borborygmus; irregularity of the bowel movement, itching of the anus, anorexia, nausea, vomiting offensive breath; while reflexly they may produce vertigo, headache, inequality of the pupils, eclampsia, chorea, and muscular spasms. The patient often complains of itching of the nose, and digs the fingers into the nostrils. He often is emaciated, pallid and has dark rings about the eyes. The worms may occupy the whole lumen of the bowel and give rise to intestinal obstruction. They wander about and may close the ductus choledoctus or pass through the stomach, esophagus, and have been known to pass during sleep into the larynx and be the cause of death. They have been found in intestinal perforation, appendiceal and perineal abcesses.

Ascaris Lumbricoides – (Remedies)	
Cina	Is of service in children when the pupils are dilated, the face is pale and there are dark rings about the eyes. The child grinds its teeth during sleep, picks and bores at its nose, and cries out during sleep.
Mercurius	Has been of service when the general symptoms call for it.
Naphthalin	Has been employed and should be studied
Santonin	Is indicted in many cases when the presence of the worm has been demonstrated. The symptoms are similar to those of cina
Also study Ant,Crud., Stannum and Spigelia	

ACUTE PERITONITIS

Definition: This is an acute inflammation of the peritoneum.

Aetiology: It is the result of wounds, bruises, and perforation of the stomach, duodenum, and small intestines, of the appendix, and the colon in malignant diseases. It results from rupture of hydrated cysts and of abscess of the various organs. The pathogenic germs that give rise to peritonitis are *bacilli coli communis, streptococci, staphyloccocipneumonococci and tubercule bacilli.*

Pathology: In the early stages the peritoneum is roughened and congested. The intestines are distended with gas. In a short time there is an inflammatory exudates on the surface of the peritoneum. This may consist of fibrin only, or serum and fibrin, pus or bloody serum, especially peritoneum. This may consist of fibrin only, or serum and fibrin, or pus or bloody serum, especially if due to an external wound. The coils of intestine are more or less adherent to one another. In cases of perforation, carcinoma and rupture of the uterus, the serum is mixed with septic material and the odor is foul. The amount of fluid varies. In long standing cases the adhesions become dense bands of tissue. In the circumscribed form the adhesions may wall off collections of pus or fluid.

Symptoms: There is an acute abdominal pain with tympanites, nausea, vomiting, constipation and elevation of temperature. The pulse is small, rapid and tense. The face is drawn and the expression is anxious, the breathing is shallow, rapid and of the thoracic type. The abdominal pain and tenderness are so intense that the patient dreads the slightest movement or pressure. The thighs are flexed on the abdomen to relax the abdominal parieties. The body is often covered with a cold sweat and collapse may be present. Should pus form, there will be rigors and hectic fever. If the process is putrid, death speedily results from septic intoxication.

Treatment: The patient should be kept quiet in bed. All pressure should be removed from the abdomen. The diet should consist of nothing but fluids. External applications, either in the form of a poultice or ice bag, should be used, according as the patient prefers. Heat may be applied in the form of a hot water bag, or a flaunel wrung out of hot water and covered with oil silk, or by a flax seed poultice, changed often and kept hot by means of oil silk.

ACUTE PERITONITIS: Remedies	
Aconite	This remedy should be studied in the early history of those cases in which the attack is the result of exposure and cold. The skin is dry and hot, the pulse is full, hard and rapid, the respirations are rapid and the temperture is high. The patient is anxious and restless; there is great thirst with vomiting. The urine is scanty and of a dark red colour. The abdomen is swollen burning and hot. There are sharp cutting pains through the abdomen.
Ars. Alb.	Should be carefully compared with Veratrum Album. The pains are violent and colicky. There is the sensation of burning and thirst and the general symptoms that should lead to its selection

Continued...

Belladonna	When this remedy is indicated the pulse is full and strong. There is much throbbing of the carotids. The face is flushed, the eye seems to protrude and the pupils are dilated. The abdomen is distended, painful and the patient complains of burning, cutting colicky pains which are worse from the slightest motion, or pressure. When this remedy fails to give the desired result, **Atropine** should be compared
Bryonia	Should be studied when serous effusion has taken place. There are stitching, lancinating pains in the bowels which are rendered worse on motion. The patient is thirsty and desires large quantities of water. The mouth, lips and tongue are very dry. The tongue has a white coating. The bowels are constipated and the patient complains of nausea when compelled to move.
Cantharis	Is indicated in cases that are attended with violent burning and cutting pains in the abdomen and extensive tympanites. There is great prostration and painful urination
Colocynthis	Is indicted in cases characterized by stinging, lancinating, burning pains in the abdomen which distended and tympanitic. The patient complains of violent, distressing pains during stool. The pulse is small and rapid. The extremities are cold. Enteritis may be associated with peritonitis.
Sulphur	Fills a place and is indicated in these cases when another remedy, although indicated, has not caused absorption of the fluid. In these cases there is a lack of reaction, recovery is not taking place, and the patient complains of great weakness. If a hectic fever is present, or if ulceration is taking place, the use of this remedy is but a loss of time.
If suppuration takes place and drainage is established, Silicea, Hepar Sulph and Calcarea Sulph should be studied.	

AILMENTS OF LIVER

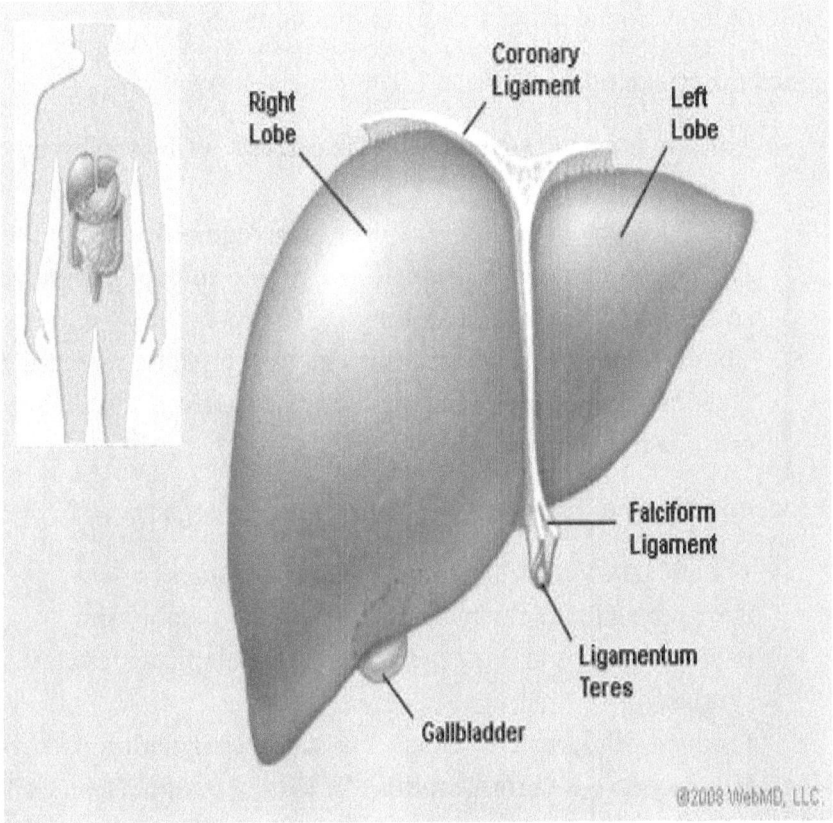

FRONT VIEW OF THE LIVER WITH ANOTOMY

The liver is a large, meaty organ that sits on the right side of the belly. Weighing about 3 pounds, the liver is reddish-brown in colour and feels rubbery to the touch. Normally you can›t feel the liver, because it is protected by the rib cage. The liver has two large sections, called the right and the left lobes. The gallbladder sits under the liver, along with parts of the pancreas and intestines. The liver and these organs work together to digest, absorb, and process food.

The liver's main job is to filter the blood coming from the digestive tract, before passing it to the rest of the body. The liver also detoxifies chemicals and metabolizes drugs. As it does so, the liver secretes bile that ends up back in the intestines. The liver also makes proteins important for blood clotting and other functions.

Various functions of the liver

- Various functions of the liver are carried out by the liver cells or hepatocytes.
- The liver produces and excretes bile, required for dissolving fats. Some of the bile drains directly into the duodenum, and some is stored in the gallbladder
- The liver performs several roles in carbohydrate metabolism: gluconeogenesis (the formation of glucose from certain amino acids, lactate or glycerol)

Glycogenolysis (the formation of glucose from glycogen)

- The breakdown of insulin and other hormones
- Is responsible for the mainstay of protein metabolism.
- Performs several roles in lipid metabolism: cholesterol synthesis
- Produce triglycerides (fats) Produces coagulation factors I (fibrinogen), II (prothrombin), V, VII, IX, X and XI, as well as protein C, Protein S and antithrombin.
- Breaks down hemoglobin, creating metabolites that are added to bile as pigment
- Breaks down toxic substances and most medicinal products in a process called drug metabolism. This sometimes results in toxication, when the metabolite is more toxic than its precursor and converts ammonia to urea.
- Stores a multitude of substances, including glucose in the form of glycogen, vitamin B12, iron, and copper.
- In the first trimester fetus, the liver is the main site of red blood cell production. By the 32nd weeks of gestation, the bone marrow has almost completely taken over that task.

- Responsible for immunological effects; the reticuloendothelial system of the liver contains many immunologically active cells, acting as a 'sieve' for antigens carried to it via the portal system.

HEPATALGIA: Hepatic Colic – Remedies	
Aconite	Violent inflammatory fever, with stitches in the region of the liver; pressure and constriction in hepatic region, with oppression of breathing; intolerable pain; jaundice present or not; moaning, tossing about, anguish and dread of death.
Aurum Met	HEPATIC CONGESTION CONSECUTIVE TO CARDIAC DISEASE, with burning and cutting in right hypochondrium, ending in cirrhosis and fatty degeneration with dropsy. Chronic hepatitis, with suicidal melancholy, averse to motion; feels stupid; jaundice with pain in liver and pit of stomach; greenish-brown urine; foul breath and putrid taste, constipation or stools of a graying or ashy-white colour. **Covers HYPERTROPHY OF LIVER, engorgement also**
Ars. alb.	Painful bloatedness in right hypochondrium, with burning pain, pain in hepatic region on pressure, stitches in right hypochondrium, extending to gastric region, ending aas violent pressure over whole abdomen, vomiting of black masses, black stools, burning heat of the skin, very quick pulse, anxiousness and restlessness, performation into the stomach or intestines.
Baptisia	PERIHEPATITIS with sharp stitches in right hypochondrium, < from any motion,> when lying on right side, pain under the right shoulder blade, swelling of swelling of the liver, bitter taste in mouth, yellow-coated tongue; stools either hard, dry and brown, or papescent and profuse, with colic, stools sometimes have odour hesse; intolerance of vegetable food; patient cannot bear heat of sun; < in summer, fuleness and bloadtedness of abdomen with sensation as if a stone or heavey weight were lying clogged in stomach; great thirst. Cases spoiled by Mer. Dul.

Continued...

HEPATALGIA: Hepatic Colic – Remedies	
Bryonia	(Cover HEPATITIS also) PERIPHEPATITIS/HEPATITIS – with sharp stitches in right hypochondrium < from any motion, > when lying on right side, pain under the right shoulder blade, swelling of the liver, bitter taste in mouth, yellow-coated tongue; stools either hard, and brown, or papascent and profuse with colic; stools sometimes have odour of old cheese; intolerance of vegetable food; patient cannot bear heat of sun: < in summer; fullness and bloatedness of abdomen with sensation as if a stone or heavy weight were lying clogged in stomach; great thirst. Cases spoiled by Merc. dul. (Cover Abcess of Liver)
Laurocerasus	WASTING AWAY OF LIVER (Phos), NUTMEG LIVER; sticking pain in liver, with pressure; distension of liver, pain as if as abscess would burst; burning or coldness in stomach and abdomen; constipation or diarrhoea; rapid sinking of the vital forces.
Merc.sol	(Cover ABCESS OF LEVER/HEPATITIS/also) LIVER ENLARGED AND OFTEN INDURATED; dirty, yellowish-white coating of tongue, which takes imprint of teeth; scorbutic symptoms; gums ulcerate and become spongy, foetid breath; jaundiced hue of skin and conjunctiva; liver sore to touch; abdomen tympanic and swollen; cannot lie on right side, stools clavey from absence of bile or yellowish-green, bilious passed with much tenesmus, and followed by a never-get-done feeling; rush of blood to head; sleeplessness from itching without eruption; mental depression, emaciation and Cover HYPERTROPHY OF LIVER, engorgement
Nux Vom.	(Cover ABCESS OF LEVER/HEPATITIS also) HEPATC AFFECTION IN GOOD LIVERS, in alcoholic excess and after allopathic dosing. Liver swollen, hard and sensitive to pressure of clothing; jaundice provoked by violent anger, abuse of quinine, with attacks of faintness, leaving him sick and weak, haemorrhoidal colic or from gastric and bilious derangements, with sudden, severe pain in right side; stitches in hepatic region, < from contact or motion.

Pulsitilla	Cover ABCESS OF LEVER/HEPATITIS also) Darting, tensive pains in hepatic region; sticking pains, particularly when walking, feeling of lassitude in hypochondria; frequent attacks of anguish, especially at night, with diarrhoea; greenish or slimy stools; bitter taste; oppression in chest and pressure at stomach.
HEPATICA REMEDIES	
Chelidonium	upto sharp stitching pains, shooting from liver down into the stomach or down into the back from posterior part of liver; MARKED PAIN UNDER THE ANGLE OF RIGHT SCAPULA, even going through the chest like a rivet; abdomen distended and sensitive to pressure; rigors in the evening, awakes in the Abdominal plethora from simple congestion to positive inflammation, soreness morning perspiring with many unremembred dreams of sleepless from headache, either continuous sharp frontal or neuralgic, in right temple and eye-brow painful throbbing in occiput; anxiety tightness, and pains in right side during inhalation, as if constricted by a girdle and cannot be expanded; attacks of rigor in the evening; irregular palpitation of heart; pain in hepatic region, > by eating; diarrhoea and constipation alternating, stools clay-coloured or yellowish great weariness and anorexia; desire for milk or acids. **Covers HYPERTROPHY OF LIVER, engorgement also**
China	subcutaneous ulceration, < from touch and very sensitive to pressure; swollen, hard liver, tympanitic abdomen, wants to belch, eructations afford no relief; gastro-duodenal catarrh, headache, bitter taste, yellowish skin, < at night and after eating; bleeding piles burning and itching, with great debility, constipation, stool difficult, even when soft or profuse, painless black, green, often offensive after diarrhoea.

Continued...

Calcarea carb	Pressure in hepatic region with every step when walking; stitches during and after stooping; ENLARGEMENT AND INDURATION OF LIVER, se3nsitive to pressure in epigastrium and abdomen, which is distended and hard; cold feet at night in bed.
Lachesis	ENLARGED LIVER OF DRUNKARDS, GOING ON TO A LOW GRADE OF SYMPTOMS with inflammation and abcess of liver, jaundis, tenderness on pressure all the time (Lyc. only after a meal), intolerance of clothing deep throbbing on right side. Liver complaints at the climax, after ague, from syphilis. Pain as if something had lodged in the right side, with stinging pains; much flatulence, palpitations, pain when coughing as from an ulcerated spot, constant tormenting urging in anus, but no stool follows, or excessively offensive stools, < in spring; gastric pains decreasing during eating and returning again after one or two hours, aching pain in shin bones; mental depression. **(Covers also ABCESS OF LIVER)**
Leptandra	Dull aching in right hypochondrium in region of gall-bladder and also in posterior portion of liver, accompanied by soreness, burning distress in and about liver, often spreading to stomach and abdomen; drowsiness and despondency; diarrhoea, STOOLS BLACK AS PITCH WITH BURNING, COLICKY PAINS AT THE NAVEL, griping continuing after stool; vomiting of bile with burning distress and occasionally clay-coloured stools; urine of a dark colour; much soreness of head and eyeballs, frequent chilliness along the spine; pain in left shoulder and arm.

Lycopodium	Cirrhosis of liver with ascites, especially in drunkards; GIN-LIVER; tongue coated sour, putrid taste in the morning on rising; hunger, but a few mouthfuls of food fill him up to the throat, quickly followed by hunger again; distress in stomach immediately after eating; tension in hypochondria after a meal, as from a cord, cannot stretch or stand upright, very sensitive to touch; flatulence tends rather upword than downward; great fermentation of bowels and ineffectual urging to stool, and after stool feeling as if great quantity remained unpassed; cold feet, or one foot cold, the other warm; chronic hepatitis with tendency to hepatic abscess; liver complaint after mortification. **Covers HYPERTROPHY OF LIVER, engorgement**
Nitric Acid	Chronic derangements, LIVER ENORMOUSLY ENLARGED; jaundice with clay-coloured stools; cadaverous smell from mouth, bloody saliva; excessive physical irritability and weakness.
Podophylum	TORPOR HEPATITIS; CHRONIC HEPATITIS, costiveness, jaundice, constantly rubbing and stroking hypochondrium with hands, fullness in right hypochondrium, hyperaemia of the liver with flatulence, pain and soreness, great irritability of liver and eccessive secretion of bile, twisting pain in right hypochondrium with sensation of heat there, jaundice, with gall-stones; pain from region of stomach towards gall-blader, with excessive nausea, with constipation and diarrhoea. POLYCHOLIA.

Continued...

HEPATICA REMEDIES	
Sepia	FUNCTIONAL DERANGEMENT OF LIVER, often proceeded by myfraine or wandering articular affections with profuse sweats; constant aching pain in right side of abdomen, extending, when violent, to chest and back, with oppression of breathing, distress and aching in right shoulder and scapula; cheeks flushed; forehead and conjunctiva yellow, also around mouth, and yellow or red saddle over bridge of nose down cheeks; IRREGULAR YELLOW PATHCES ON PAGE; tendency to perspire,especially between scapulae, mammae and under axillae; occipital headache; gastroses, tongue flbby and indented, no appetite or easily satisfied, < from acids or fats; flatulence; stools bright-yellow or of an ashy colour; urine scantyand loae with urates; lassitude, atony of connective tissue and relaxation of bloodvessels; TISSUE TORPIITY RELIEVED BY EXERCISE WHICH HURRIES ON THE BLOOD; feels < when awaking, when sitting, always > by a good walk, but scending painful;> from eructations, with desire to pass flatus downwod, < in close rooms, in foggy weather, during nursing; pain in hypochondria more tolerable when lying on painful side; hepatic neuralgia with great depression of spirits, frequent stitches under right ribs. **(Cover Abcess of liver)**
HYPERTROPHY OF LIVER	
Agaricus	Congested, enlarged liver; sensation of pain and drawing in right hypochondrium, as if the liver had increased in weight and dragged at its ligaments; sharp stitches as from needles in the hepatic region; dull stitches during breathing; pain in stomach and liver, burning from acidity.
Chionanthus	HYPERTROPHY OF LIVER: constipation, stools clay-coloured, skin and urine jaundiced, great emaciation; soreness in region of liver, quick, weak pulse. Chronic jaundice, recurring every summer, urine almost black, after abuse of mercurials.

Magn. mur	ENLARGED LIVER OF CHILDREN, who are punny in their growth and rachitic. Pressing pains in enlarged hard liver when walking, or touching it, < when lying on right side; regurgitation when walking; knotty stools, like sheep-dung or diarrhoea, tongue large, coated yellow, takes imprint of teeth; dyspnoea and palpitations, < when quiet and > from moving about; oedema pedum; uterine diseases and indurated os; hemorrhagic diathesis; frequent fits, hysterical uterine and abdominal cramps, extending into thighs.
Ptelea trif:	Spains in the right hypochondrium
Sulphur	HYPERTROPHY OF LIVER, engorgement/HEPATITIS: Swelling and hardness of the liver; stitches hardness of the liver, thirst; insomnia or sleep in cat naps; constipation; haemorrhoids; dyspepsia of drunkards.

ABCESS OF LIVER	
Belladonna	Acute pain in hepatic region, worse from pressure, breathing, coughing and lying upon the right side, extending upward towards shoulder and neck, congestion of head; getting dark before eyes, fainting and giddiness, bloatedness of pit of stomach; tension across epigastrium, agonizing, tossing about; sleeplessness, or wanting to sleep, with inability to do so.
Silicea	Throbbing ulcerative pain in hepatic region, worse from touch or walking; ABCESSOF LIVER; hardness, distention of liver, beating soreness in liver, worse on motion, when lying on right side; burning or throbbing in pit of stomach; disgust for warm food, desires only cold things; painless diarrhoea, with exhaustion or constipation from inactivity of rectum.

PASSIVE STAGNATION OP LIVER; NUTMEG LIVER; Remedies 1st Grade: Carb.Veg. Lycopodium, Nat.Mur. and Nux.Vom. 2nd Grade: Ipecac. Nux Mosch. Phos. Veratrum alb. 3rd grade: Ars. Lachesis., Leptandria., Sulph. – Notes on Remedies available in the above list.

Continued...

CIRRHOSIS HEPATIS: Interstitial hepatitis: granulated liver: 1ˢᵗ Grade: Arg. Nit., *Aur.Met.* Bryonia., Carduus mar., *Iod* Lach. Lyc. Merc.sol. Natr.Mur. Nux.Vom. *Phos.* Plumb. – – **2ⁿᵈ Grade:** Carb.Veg., Puls. **3ʳᵈ Grade:** Ars. Chel., China., Leptandria., Nitr. Acid., Magn. Mur. Selen., milk diet especiallydueing first stages
PYLEPHLEBITIS: inflammation of portal vein; the same as CIRRHOSIS prrenata
HEPATITIS DIFFUSA, acute yellow atrophy of the liver: **Remedies:** Aconite, Bell. Bry., Calc.carb., Digitalis, Ipecac., Leptandria., during Typhoid also: Ars..., china., Crotalus., Phosphorous, Phos.acid., Sulphuric acid (haemorrhage)
HEPAR ADIPOSUM: fatty liver; **COLLOID LIVER,** waxy liver: Arg. Nit. Bell., Carb.an., Hydrastis, Lyco., Sep. sil.
CARCINOMA HEPATITIS: Ars. Bell. Carb. Animolis., Hydrastis., Lyco., Sep. sil.

Gallbladder:

Gallbladder is a pear shaped organ that stores about 50 ml of bile (or "gall") until the body needs it for digestion. The gallbladder is about 7–10cm long in humans and is dark green in appearance due to its contents (bile), not its tissue. It is connected to the liver and the duodenum by the biliary tract.

It is connected to the main bile duct through the gallbladder duct (cystic duct). The main biliary tract runs from the liver to the duodenum, and the cystic duct is effectively a "cul de sac", serving as entrance and exit to the gallbladder. The surface marking of the gallbladder is the intersection of the midclavicular line (MCL) and the trans pyloric plane, at the tip of the ninth rib. The blood supply is by the cystic artery and vein, which runs parallel to the cystic duct. The cystic artery is highly variable, and this is of clinical relevance since it must be clipped and cut during a cholecystectomy.

Has an epithelial lining characterized by recesses called Aschoff's recesses, which are pouches inside the lining. Under the epithelium there is a layer of connective tissue, followed by a muscular wall that contracts in response to cholecystokinin, a peptide hormone synthesized in the duodenum.

The gallbladder stores bile, which is released when food containing fat enters the digestive tract, stimulating the secretion of cholecystokinin (CCK). The bile emulsifies fats and neutralizes acids in partly digested food. After being stored in the gallbladder, the bile becomes more concentrated than when it left the liver, increasing its potency and intensifying its effect on fats, anal canal and peristaltic waves propel the feacas out of the rectum. The internal and external sphincters of the anus allow the feaces to be passed by muscles pulling the anus up over the existing feaces.

GAL BLADDER – CHOLOCYSTITIS (Inflammation of Gall – Bladder)

SYMPTOMS: Constant and persisting abdominal flatulency. Whenever there is constant flatulency and no relief with any other flatulent remedies, suspect about the disease in gall – bladder.

Remedies:

- Chelidonium ... Stones
- Cholesterinum ... Stones
- China – Cardusmar ... Swelling
- Hydrastis, Phosphorous... Inflammation
- Calc. carb.... Gall-bladder colic – Specific

Gall stones – How they are formed?

When from various causes, liver is unable to produce the bile salts in sufficient quantity, there is high cholesterol condition in the blood and bile, with eventual deposition of cholesterol and formation of gall-stones may be the result. Normal individuals can eat food containing cholesterol because more bile salts are produced by the liver and hold the cholesterol in solution, *and with other individuals the capacity is defective.* The foods which increase the cholesterol content of the blood are: **egg yolk, butter, creamy liver, kidney, Pancreas, brain and meat fats.**

Gall Stones (Remedies)	
Aconite	Is indicated in the very early stages of the diseases if there has been an exposure to cold or dampness, or if the perspiration has been checked. The stools are green, scanty, loose, and frequent and are attended with tenesmus. The patient is restless, anxious and the temperature is above normal.
Ars. Alb.	When the stools are watery, mucous or blood. The patient is weak, exhausted and pale, and complain of faintness, rapid exhaustion, and burning in the rectum. The cheeks are sunken and there is great restlessness and exhaustion after the stools.
Aloes	Indicated when there is pain and rumbling in the bowels before the stools, which may be involuntary. At times the stools pass without any exertion or escape with flatus. A feeling of insecurity, so that the patient is not certain whether it is flatus or feacal matter that is to escape. There is much flatus with each stools, and following each stools there is a sensation as though more remained in the rectum.
Belladonna	During the early stage, when the pupils are dilated and the carotids throbbing. The stools are small, frequent and involuntary, and are followed by tenesmus. The patient is sleepy but restless, and starts up from sleep suddenly. There is constant pressing towards the anus and genitals as if everything would press out. Pains come and go suddenly.
Cuprum Ars.	In cases characterised by frequent discharges and sharp cutting, colicky pains. Stools are usually tinged with green and with an offensive odour. They are usually accompanied by vomiting.
Croton Tig.	Stools are forcible, "coming out like a shot, yellow and watery. Condition is aggravated from the taking of food or drink.

Chamomilla	For patients who are irritable, peevish and oversensitive to pain. he stools are yellow-green and watery. It is frequently useful in diarrheic attacks that accompany dentition.
Calcarea Carb	Great chillines during attack; darting pain from right to left, with profuse sweat, abdominal spasms and colic, cutting colic in epigastrium, has to bend double, clench hands, writhe with agony.
Carduus mar	Haepatic region sensitive to pressure; crawling sensation, like passage of a small body through a narrow canal, on posterior side of liver from right to left and extending to pit of stomach.
Chelidonium	Chill with intense pain in region of gall-bladder quickly extending down and across navel into intestines; with vomiting amnd clay-coloured stools; pain from liver shooting towards back and shoulder.
Chenopodium	Severe pain in the region of the lower inner angle of the right scapula running into the chest; cold feet up to the knees; tired legs and knees, constipation, stools like sheep-dung, hard and knotty.
China	Obstruction in gall-bladder with colic, periodic recurrence, yellow skin and conjunctiva, constipation, with dark-greenish scybala; sensitive to least pressure
Chionanthus	Gall-stone colic; sensation like a string tied around intestines in umbilical region, every once in awhile it is suddenly drawn tight and then gradually loosened; somewhat > by lying on stomach and abdomen.
Dioscorea	Cutting pains, changing location and radiating; much flatulency.
Ferr. Phos	Should be remembered in weak, delicate, anaemic subjects when the attack is produced by exposure. There is slight fever. Stools are undigested, copious, watery, sudden and painful and may be accompanied with vomiting.

Continued...

Gelsimium	In cases when sudden depressing emotion, fright, grief, bad news, patient desires to be quiet and alone and is drowsy. The pulse is soft and flowing and there is a slight fever.
Gambogia	Desire for stools is sudden and passed with one great effort, after which there is a sensation of great relief as if some irritating substance has been removed. There is great rumbling of gas in the bowels. The stools consist of yellow or green watery material.
Iris Vers	Cases in which there is vomiting of bilious material. Yellowish green colour stools containing much bile. They leave the anus excoriated and raw. The attacks are worse during hot weather and are attended with headache.
Lycopodium	Violent gall-stone colic; hepatic region sensitive to cobtact; heartburn, waterbrash; constipation and flatulency.
Merc. Dul	Indicated in cases in which the stools are preceded by colic and is followed by tenesmus. The stools are slimy, bloody, acrid and burning
Nux Mosch.	Enlarged liver, bloody stools; weight about liver; pressure as from asharp or stones; swollen feeling, must bend double
Podophylum	Jaundice with gall-stones pain from region of stomach towards region of gall-bladder, with excessive nausea, constantly rubbing towards region of gall-bladder, with nausea; constantly rubbing and stroking hypochondrium with hands; alternate constipation and diarrhoea.
Silicea	Hepatic abcess, with throbbing, ulcerative pain, from touch or walking; constipation, stool large and expulsion difficult.
Varatrum Alb.	Should be remembered in cases in which the stools are watery, sudden, involuntary, painful and copious. The body is blue and old, the face indicates collapse. There is copious vomiting and a cold perspiration is on the forehead.

RECTUM/ANUS

Pains – Inflammation – Proctitis Proctalgia – Constipation – Prolapsus Ani/Prolapsus Infantum

Anus is situated between the buttocks, posterior to the perineum. It has two anal **sphincters**, one internal, the other external. These hold the anus closed until defecation occurs. One **sphincter consists of smooth muscle** and its **action is involuntary**; the other consists of **striated muscle** and its action is **voluntary**. In many animals, the anus is surrounded by anal sacs. Role of the anus is when the rectum is full, the increase in intra-rectal pressure forces the walls of the anal canal apart allowing the feacal matter to enter the canal. The rectum shortens as material is forced into the Anus

RECTUM/ANUS AND REMEDIES	
Belladonna	Catarrhal inflammation, constriction of anus – Pressing and urging towards anus and genitals, alternating with contractions of the anus; spasmodic constriction of anus, as in dysentery.
Causticum	Fruitless urging to stool, with faintness; with anxiety and red face. constriction of anus
Cocculus	Tenesmus recti after stool, with faintness; lessend peritistalis, Constriction of anus.
Ignatia	Proctalgia, contraction, with cutting, shooting paging, <after stool, symptoms irregular, fitful, as in hysteria. During stool erection erection of penis. Constriction of anus.
Kali bich	Sensation of a plug; diarrhoea of brown, frothy water, spurting out in early morning and followed by tenesmus ani. Constriction of anus.
Lachesis	Tormenting urging in rectum, but on account of constriction of anus it becomes so painful he must desist; protruding piles with constricted anus. Catarrhal inflammation of rectum.
Mezerium	After the anus is constricted around the protruding rectum.

Continued...

RECTUM/ANUS AND REMEDIES	
Natrum Mur	Sensation of contraction in rectum during stool, faeces tear the anus; frequent ineffectual urging; spasmodically constriction of anus.
Nitric acid	Sticking in rectum as from splinter; constriction during stool and lasting for hours afterwards; rectum feels as if torn.
Opium	Obstinate constipation; anus spasmodically closed, during colic; inactivity of bowels, stools consisting of hard, round, black balls; flatulency from inertia. Constriction of anus.
Plumbum	Retraction of abdomen; marked spasm of contraction of sphincter ani; urging to stool; and sensation as if a string were drawing the anus up into the rectum; faeces hard and dry from absorption of their moisture. Constriction of anus.

CONSTIPATION

AETIOLOGY:

This prevails in certain families. It may be dependent upon a false modesty of some who, instead of training the bowels to evacuate themselves, suppress the desire. This is especially true of girls while at school, while upon visits or at summer resorts. A diet that leaves but little residue is another cause. The prolonged employment of cathartics results in intestinal paresis. In other cases there is intestinal dilatation that is responsible for the constipation, while in others it is dependent upon a lack of nourishment, and as a result there is not enough residue to cause the irritation and reflex act necessary to evacuation of the bowels. Lack of exercise, an insufficient amount of fluid, an improper diet, as an excess of milk and cheese, are other causes. In other cases irregular habits and postponement of defecation, hemorrhoids, rectal ulcers, all favour constipation.

Symptoms: This depend upon the acuteness of the condition. In mild cases there is headache, coated tongue, gripping pain, and occasionally attacks of vomiting; with these there is a passage of a small quantity of feacal matter.

In more pronounced cases the symptoms develop slowly and consist of headache, a coated tongue and abdominal discomfort. An examination of the abdomen shows the colon to be impacted, especially in the right iliac region, at times also the left and the flexures of the colon. The mass may be tender, it is irregular in shape and can be moulded by pressure and is completely removed by enema. Intestinal colic may occur when there has been prolonged irregularity of the diet with neurosis. In many cases the feaces are but partially evacuated and old, inodorous faecal matter remains in the colon. In the aged especially, diarrhea may co-exist as a result of the irritation of the retained faecal matter.

Treatment: Each case must be studied separately for its etiology, and the diet and the patient's habits considered. In beginning the management of these cases the bowels should be thoroughly cleared of all matter by high injections of sweet oil and the internal administration of olive oil, two ounces twice a day. Following this it is advisable to use massage or vibratory massage, beginning mildly and increasing as the patient can endure it. The treatments should be applied to the affected points only.

The diet also must be regulated. The patient must drink a sufficient amount of fluid; this may embrace water, milk, cream and fruit juices, but they should be taken till atleast three pints of urine is passed in twenty-four hours. The diet should be such that it contains much residue, especially cellulose. Fruits should be taken three times a day. Tea and coffee are not to be allowed. Massage should be confined to the line of the colon. Exercise is beneficial in the majority of cases. In some weak, delicate women, who suffer from ovarian or uterine irtitation, exercise appears to aggravate rather than improve the condition.

In certain cases a relaxation of the muscles of the abdomen or a pendulous abdomen is the cause of the constipation. In these cases a well-fitting abdominal bandage or passive movements of the abdominal muscles are of service. The daily use of light dumb bells, bending backward and forward from the hips, rotating to the body from the hips, horseback riding, golf and tennis are to be recommended. Regular timings to be strictly adhered to.

Ulcers and haemorrhoids are responsible for constipation which should be corrected. Massage may be practiced by the patient or by an attendant. The movements should commence in the splenic flexure of the colon, that the transverse colon may be unloaded. Following this the movements should be commenced at the ceacum that the whole length of the colon may be embraced in the treatment. Gentle percussion or vibration over the line of the colon is beneficial. The rolling of a five pound shot over the abdomen is also employed

CONSTIPATION REMEDIES	
Aesculus Hip	Should be studied in those cases in which there are haemorrhoids. The stools are hard, dry and difficult to evacuate. There is a sensation as of sticking in the rectum and severe lumbo – sacral backache.
Aethusa Cyn	Most obstinate constipation, with feeling as if all action of the bowels had been lost; thirst with total loss of appetite for every kind of ailment; intolerance of milk; soreness and painfulness in both hypochondria; head confused, brain feels bound up; morose and cross.
Agaricus	Obstinate constipation following diarrhoea in old spirit drinkers, who are full of nervous symptoms, as loss of appetite, insomonia cirrhotic liver; painful straining in rectum before stool, during stool colic and passing of flatus; mucous haemorrhoids with slime oozing out without the stool; headache > after stool; delirium tremens.

Aloe	Constant urging to stool, passing small quantities; sometimes only a few drops of blood; CONSTIPATION OF PERSONS WHO LIVE TO EAT; constipation of old people with abdominal plethora; suitable to hypochondriacs and to bookworms, with pituitous state of stomach and bowels; heat, soreness and heaviness of rectum; heaviness in pelvis and dull, heavy sensation in sacral region, < while sitting and >by motion; urging as with diarrhoea, only hot flatus passes, with sensation as if a plug were wedged between symphysis and coccyx, INVOLUNTARY, UNNOTICED HARD STOOL.
Alumen	Evacuations hard and knotty, discharged with great difficulty and at LONG INTERVALS, once or twice a week, sick headache in the morning; frequent cramps in pit of stomach and vomiting with some retching. LONG-LASING PAIN IN RECTUM AFER EACH STOOLS; painful bleeding piles, with aching in anus; deathlike fainting spells, with loss of all faculties.
Ambra grisea	Frequent ineffectual desire for stool which makes her very anxious, and AT THIS TIME THE PRESENCE OF OT HER PERSONS BECOMES UNBEARABLE; sensate ion of coldness in abdomen. Melancholy with sad weeping, great weakness, loss of muscular power, pain in small of back an constipation; especially during child bed.
Alumina	TORPOR OF RECTUM. No desire for and no ability to pass stool till there is a large accumulation; disposition when at stool to grasp the seat tightly, perspiration breaks out, the patient almost despairs of effecting a discharge; nausea nd faintness, nervouis exhaustion, tremulous weakness of lower extremities, chilliness during and after stool. Inactivity of rectum, EVEN A SOFT STOOL, LIKE PUTTY, AND STICKING TO ANUS, REQUIRES GREAT STRAINING, urine passes while straining at stool; stool sometimes in the shape of laurel-berries; < afternoon, periodical, in warm room, travelling; > in fresh air, passes stool better standing (caust.). Often suitable to the aged and infirm and to nursing children; ailments from lead poisoning (Op).

Continued...

CONSTIPATION REMEDIES	
Amm.Mur	Hard stools, rumbling to pieces when defaecating, requiring great efforts to expel them, followed by soft stool; the FAECES ARE COVERED WITH A GLAIRY TOUGH MUCUS, and are accompanied by a discharge of a quantitiy of mucus and much flatus; piles after suppression of leucorrhea.
Anacardium	Frequent tenesmus for many days, without being able to pass anything; great urgent desire for stool, but on sitting down the desire immediately passes off without an evcacuation; the rectum seems to be powerless, with a sensation as if plugged up; frequent bleeding from the anus when at the stool; headache with sensation as if there were a plug in the head, with mental irritability and propensity to swear.
Amm.Carb	Costiveness on account of hardness of faeces, difficult to expel, with headache, protrusion of haemorrhoids after stool, with long-lasting pains, cannot walk; listless and lethargic.
Amm.Mur	Hard stools, rumbling to pieces when defaecating, requiring great efforts to expel them, followed by soft stool; the FAECES ARE COVERED WITH A GLAIRY TOUGH MUCUS, and are accompanied by a discharge of a quantitiy of mucus and much flatus; piles after suppression of leucorrhea.
Ant. Crud.	Alternate constipation and diarrhoea, especially of old people; difficult, hard stool, faeces too large; constive with incarcerated flatus and colic; constiveness in the heat of summer; constipation during child-bed; suicidal despondency, anxiousness of mind and sensitiveness to sound; frontal headache and dizziness on ascending st airs; tongue while, complete loss of appetit e; gulping up of fluid, tasting of the ingesta, nausea and vomiting. Children's stools white, dry, with hard lumps of curd.

Apis mell	Chronic constipation. Feeling in anus as if it were stuffed full, with heat and throbbing in rectum. Large, hard, difficult stools, only once or twice a week; stinging pains and sensation in abdomen as from something tight, which would break if much effort were made.
Arnica	No urging; inactivity of rectum, stool INSUFFICIENT, hard, much starining, with headache, head hot; feels full all over and unfit for business; belching. After a blow on epigastrium, from concussion, overexertion.
Ars.Alb	Constipation with inability to drink cold water and oain in bowels.
Asafoetida	Obstinate constipation, with abdominal and haemorrhoidal cramps; constant ineffectual to stool, with violent pressing towards the rectum and discharge of offensive flatus; only slime passes, no faeces.
Arum	Hard, knotty and large stools; costiveness worse during menses; piles with rectal catarrh.
Baptisia	Constipation, with torpor of the liver and haemorrhoids in the afternoon, very troublesome; stool very small and difficult to pass, it resembles sheep's dung, passed only by very great straining and urging; pain before stool, weakness after stool, dull lumbar headache, < walking
Baryta Carb	Obstinate constipation with apoplectic oldmen whose physical and moral forces are exhausted; stools scanty, hard and lumpy, expelled with difficulty; want of clear consciousness, second childhood.
Belladonna	No urging; plethora abdominal and spasmodic; clutching pains come quick; forehead, eyes, red; carotids throbbing; tongue coated; sour taste, eructations. Urine dark; dull and stupid. Ileus, lead colic; stools suppressed with bloated abdomen, heat of head and abundant sweat; pains in kidneys and sensation of compression in chest; fretful, indolent before stool, contended and cheerful after. From cold or suppressed perspiration, < afternoon and evening.

Continued...

Berberis	Constipation from constriction of anus; hard stool, like sheep's dung, passed only after hard straining; burning, stitching pain before, urging and after stool. Fistula recti with bilious symptoms, < when sitting; herpes aroud anus; dark, brownish-yellow face, vertigo, headache, sleepiness; dry, sticky tongue, haemorrhoids.
Bryonoia	Intestinal inactivity from perversion of gastric and hepatic functions; inertia of rectum; constipation of lying in women; costiveness during hot weather. STOOLS HARD, DARK BROWN OR BLACK, DRY AS IF BURNT, too large insize, from dryness of the alimentary tract, and passed with difficulty, attended perhaps by prolapsus of rectum and burning sensation; great dryness of tongue, mouth and lips, with thirst for large quantities of water, nausea after eating, waterbrash, vomiting, disposition to headache and to become irritable and angry. Rheumatic diathesis. Prefers cool weather; often caused by cold drinks or cold food.
Calc.carb	No urging, stools at first hard, then mushy and finally fluid, smelling like rotten eggs; involuntary, fermented, sour-smelling diarrhoea, alternating with constipation; stools looking like lumps of chalk in children during dentition, stools hard, undigested; bleeding from anus after stool; feeling of faintness; late in going to sleep; < in the morning before breakfast; in cold, wet weather; on ascending, from milk, after eating, getting wet; > after breakfast, loosening garments, rubbing.
Calc.Phos	Hard stool. With depression of mind, causing headache and vertigo in old people; hard stools with much blood, after stool buzzing in ears, with weak feeling in male sexual parts.

Carb.an	No urging, stool very hard, passed with much difficulty and streaked with blood; stool scanty and passed in pieces with difficulty; during stool pain in back and feeling across abdomen as if there were no expulsive power; thinks to defaecate, but only passes wind; constant oozing of inodorous fluid from rectum. Repugnance to greasy food; food causes distress; tiresome to eat; melancholy; head feels as if top were open, or were lifted off, or were blown to pieces, has to hold it together in damp weather.
Carbo Veg.	Ineffectual urging to stool, only wind passes with painful pressure in rectum, but feels relived by passage of flatus; tough, scanty, not properly cohering stool enveloped in mucus; sensation of complete emptines in abdomen, remaining a long time after stool.
Cascarilla	Constipation, stool hard, in pieces, covered with mucus (Graph.); constant urging, often with pain high up in rectum, gnawing pain, passes bright blood, with or without stool, in large quantities.
Causticum	Fruit less urging to stool, with anxiety and red face; dryness of rectum,with great constriction of sphincter ani and pains in rectum during stool, so that children try to keep back the evacuation; knotty, difficult stool, shining as if greased, with greasy taste in mouth, stool very small in sise and burning in anus after stool; involuntary, hard stool, < when passing wind; STOOL PASSES EASIER STANING (Alum.); pain in anus and rectum when walking, < evenings, in cold air, in clear, fine weather, from coffee, after stool; > from cold water, from warmth, in damp, wet weather. Sad, suspicious and distrustful.

Continued...

Chelidonium	With stool sensatioin as if anus were contracted; burning and cutting in rectum, with constriction of anus, alternating with itching in anus; stool like sheep's dung; great pain in hepatic and caecal regioin; gurgling in abdomen distended with flatus; frequent discharge of flatus; ICTERUS; pale, yellow face, flabby tongue, reddish urine; CONSTANT DULL PAIN UNDER LOWER AND INNER ANGLE OF RIGHT SHOULDER-BLADE; vertigo and difficult breathing after eating; alternation of diarrhoea and constipation.
China	No urging; constipation with vertigo, heat in head and tinnitus aurioum; LARGE ACCUMULATION OF FAECES, ESPECIALLY AFTER CONTINUED PURGING, with difficulty to pass them, even when soft, from inactivity of rectum; checked perspiration. Sensation of fullness in abdomen after eating, flatulency, flat taste, vomiting of sour matter; sleeplessness.
Coca erthroxylon	Constipation from inactivity of rectum; violent palpitations from incarcerated flatus, rising someties with such force that it seems as if the esophagus would be torn by it; violent bellyache with tympanitic distension of abdomen, > by discharge of inodorous flatus; can eat but little at a time.
Cocculus	No urging; hard stool every other day (Caual.) or every three or four days, passed with much difficulty; sensatioin of hollowness in stomach or abdomen; eructations, vomiting of bile; disposition to stool, but the peristaltic motion in upper intestines is wanting; sensation of numbness in limbs, < open air, > in room.
Collinsonia	Pelvic congestion; constipation during pregrancy and in connection with uterine disorders, CONGESTIVE INERTIA OF THE BOWELS, weight and pressure in rectum, with intense irritation and itching in ano; obstinate constipation with haemorrhoids, stools very sluggish and hard, light-colored, accompanied with haemorrhoids, stools very sluggish and hard, light-colored, accompanied by pain and flatulence; sensation as of sand in rectum, as if sticks or gravel had loged in lower part of rectum and anus; extreme tenderness in rectum; prolapsus ani (aesc. Hip); bowels move more evenings.

CONSTIPATION REMEDIES	
Colocynthis	Frequent urging to stools without any evacuatioins, which appears an hour later in single pieces of a stony hardness,torpor of whole-intestinal canal, acting only every other day, though the stools are not particularly hard; constipation produced by cheese; > by smoking.
Conium	Frequent or constant urging without stool; constipation following parturition, after taking milk; yellow skin; heartburn; frequent attacks of feeling sick; faint feeling after stool; vertigo when lying down and turning head; < while lying down; > when moving about, before breakfast.
Crocus	Most obstinate constipation in grown persons or children, based on venous disturbances; sensitive, long, dull stitch near left side of anus; stools contain dark stringy blood.
Euphorbium	Constipation from torpidity of bowels; hard stool, with difficult evacuation, stool like glue; violent itching of rectum during urgent desire to stool and after stool, burning sore pain around anus.
Fel.tauri & Fel. pulvis	Constipation with accumulation of flatus in intestines.
Ferrum	Constipation from intestinal atony; stools hard and difficult, followed by bacache; chronic constipation, ineffectual urging anaemia, easily flushed face and head, with cold hands and feet; pallor and sallowness with haggard features and sunken eyes often met in dyspeptic addicted to masturbation; loss of appetite, meat disagrees; eructations after eating, regurgitation of food; fullness of epigastrium and rumbling of flatulence; faeces dry; < from drinking cold water.

Continued...

Graphites	Atonic dyspepsia and constipation, with dryness of the mucous membrane of rectum and fissure ani; no great urging and no desire for stool, frequently omits the regular stools; knotty stool, THE FLATTENED LUMPS COVERED WITH MUCUS AND UNITED WITH MUCOUS THREADS; stools very large in size, or only the size of a lumbricus; a quantitity of white mucus is discharged with each stool; sensation in rectum as if much remained after stool; prolapsus recti with varices; as if retum were paralyzed; stitching, tearing and soreness in rectum during stool and for hours afterwards, < when sitting; render haemorrhoids; sleeps late in the morning; bad odor from mouth; obstructed flatus; flushes; yellow sweat, > from eructating; dryness of skin; herpetic constitution; < from all meats.
Hepar sulph	Inactivity of rectum, stool not abnormally hard, unsatisfactory, with swelling of the anus; urging to stool, but the large intestines are wanting in peristaltic action and cannot expel the faeces which are not hard, and only a portion of them can be forced out by the action of the abdominal muscles; sleep unrefeshing; acid urine; dry eruptive diseases; < in dry, clear weather, in cold air; > warmth, wrapping up head or body, in damp, wet weather. Stomach easily deranged, vomiting every morning; frequent tasteless belching. Has taken mercury to excecss (Chin.)
Hydrastis	No desire for stool, stool lumpy with or without mucus; sensation as if the bowels would move, but only wind passes; with urging to urinate; after stool pain in rectum for hours; colicky pains with sensation of goneness, faintness and heat of intestines. Constipation, caused more by slugish state of bowels in persons of sedentary habit, or from abuse of cathartics, is the cause of all other ailments.

Ignatia	Constipation in consequence of cold, or from carriage riding; prociden – tia recti during stool, which passes without much effort; violent desire for stool, more in the superior intestines and epigastrium than in the colon and anus; desire for stool keeps on a long time after faeces passed; constriction of anus after stool, < while standing; stools large or soft, but passed with difficulty.
Indium	Constipation, must strain greatly, seizing his thigh with his hands; face red, head feels as if it would burst; burning tenesmus and pain in anus after stool.
Iodium	Constipation, with ineffectual urging, > after drinkibng milk; stools hard, knotty, dark-colored. Constipation alternating with diarrhoea.
Kali bich.	Habiatual constipation, stools scanty, knotty, followed by burning and painful retraction of rectum and anus; periodical costiveness; constipation, debility, coated tongue, headache, cold extremities; sensation of a plug in anus which feels sore, making it very painful to walk.
Kreosutum	Ineffectual, painful urging to stool; faeces hard and only expelled after much straining; CONSTRICTION FROM CARCINOMATOUS TUMORS, constipation during menses; stitches in rectum, extending towards left groin.
Lachesis	STOOLS ENORMOUSLY LARGE and painful, leaving the sphincters nearly paralyzed and slow to close, with a feeling of inability to draw up the partially prolapsed anus; the anus feels closed, only single flatus are passed; stools seems to press upon anus, but nothing passes, beating in anus as from little hamers; sensation of weight, fulnes and pressure in bowels, with considerable flatus; stools offensive, even if formed; patient tired of life, especially in those who have abused alcohol; worse from abuse of mercury, liquors or narcotics; < while eating. Constipation of years' standing.

Continued...

Lycopodium	Depressed and imperfect digestion, constant sensation as if the bowels were loaded; torpor of bowels faeces hard, scanty, passed with difficulty, from constriction of the sphincter ani, and feeling as if much remained behind; much loud flatus and croaking in left hypochondrium; obstructed flatus, with pains striking from right to left; itching and tension at anus in the evening in bed; itching eruptions at anus, painful to touch; sense of fullness after eating, even very little, with drowsiness, sour vomiting; nightly restlessness; < 4 to 8 P.M. from cold food, cabbage and vegetables with husks, oysters, from wrapping up, > in company, on getting cool, after loosening garments, discharge of flatus either way, from uncovering head or body, from warm food; ADOMINAL PLETHORA, WITH CONSTIPATION IN ELDERLY PEOPLE OF THE HIGHER CLASSES, SUFFERING FROM RETARDED DEFAECATION.

CONSTIPATION REMEDIES	
Magnesia Carb	Frequent, ineffectual urging to stool, with small discharges, or only flatus passes; stitches in anus and rectum,with fruitless desire for stool; stool only every second day.
Magnesia mur	Obstruction of bowels from induration of faeces, WHICH ARE SO DRY THAT THEY CRUMBLE AS THEY PASS THE ANUS; hard, knotty; difficult passage, discharging only a very small quantity of faeces at a time like sheep's dung, covered with blood and mucus; abdomen tense, sore as if bruised, sensitive to touch, but > from pressure; pricking pain in rectum as the stool passes; aching in liver, throbbing in pit of stomach; fainting nausea, < early, after rising; ATONY OF BOWELS AND BLADDER, accumulated urine causes no urging to pass it.

Mercurius	Constipation, stool tenacious and crumbling, discharged only with violent straining; constant, ineffectual urging, <at night; prolapsus ani after stool; faeces of small shape or very large in size, leaving the anus raw and sore; < from cold air, getting warm in bed.
Nat.carb	Constipation in sad, desponding and hypochondriac persons; frequent urging, but insufficient stool with tenesmus, though the faeces are not hard; burning in eyes and urethra, with great sexual excitement; < starchy and vegetable food.
Natrum mur	Obstinate constipation, with troublesome perspiration at the slightest movement; difficult expulsion of faeces, fissuring the anus, with flow of blood,leaving a sensation of much soreness at the anus; a riping-up sensation in the anus after stool; heaviness through the pelvis and across the bladder, worse when walking about; constipation from inactivity of the rectum; irritable skin; mind depressed; stools hard, difficult, crumbling; spasms of sphincter; tendency to catarrhal affections, to eczema and other eruptions, after cold; irritability and dryness of the mucous membranes; emaciation. It rouses up the tonicity of the intestinal mucous membrane, and when the bowels are free, the mind is relieved.
Nat. sulph.	Hard, knotty stool streaked with blood, preceded and accompanied by smarting at the anus; difficult expulsion of soft stool, emission of foetid flatus in large quantities.
Nux Mosch.	Constipation for days; no desire, no urging; the rectum becomes filled and seems entirely paralyzed.
Oxalic acid	Frequent, ineffectual urging to stool, pressed by sick, distressed feeling from the navel downward, < when thinking of it. Now and then a profuse, watery, gushing diarrhoea.

Continued...

Phosphorus	Inveterate constipation with disappointing calls, the trouble being in rectum; faeces slender, long, narrow, dry, tough and hard, like a dog's, and voided with difficulty; sour vomiting with constipation; very weak and empty feeling in abdomen; much belching; emaciation; <lying on left side or back; > lying on right side, by cold food, cold water till it gets warm in stomach, then vomits it up.
Phytolacca	Habitual costiveness, especially of old people or of those of weak constitutional powers, with weak heart 's action, intermittent pulse and general relaxed muscular system. Senstion as if the bowels would not move without the aid of laxatives; feeling of fullness in abdomen before stool, while remains after stool as if all had not passed; continual inclination to stool, but often passes only foetid flatus; torpor of rectum; pains shooting from anus and lower part of rectum along perineum to the middle of penis.
Platina	Torpor of whole intestinal canal: CONSTIPATION OF EMIGRANTS OR WHILE TRAVELLING; after lead poisoning; frequent urging, with expulsion of only small portions of faeces, with great straining; after stool sensation of great weakness in abdomen, and chilliness; stool seems to stick to t he anus, like putty (Sarsap.)
Plumbum	No flatus, fissures of anus and stricture in rectum; persistent spasm of the muscular structure of the intestines; tenesmus recti, a finger passed within the sphincter is immediately grasped; sensation as if a string drew the anus up into the rectum; stools consisting of small, hard, black balls, like sheep's dung; tympany, especially of colon, resisting pressure, with colic and a sensation of being pulled from FRONT TO BACK, AS IF THE ABDOMEN NEARLY TOUCHED THE SPINE, evacuation obstructed by the conglomeration of the little balls into one mass; < at night; from pressure; from eating hot or cold food, from motion.

Podophyllum	Infantile constipation after an attack of diarrhoea, stools hard, crumbly, clayey; costiveness in persons of sedentary habits from atony of lower intestines, stools hard, dry, clauyey, crumble when passing; with great straining and causing prolapsed of rectum with a mucuos discharge impaired digestion; headache; foetid flatus; frequent urination; pain and weakness in back; <mornings.
Pulsitilla	Chronic constipation from irregular menstruation; inactivity of intestines, whether stool is hard or soft, with painful urging to stool and backache; nauseous, bad taste in the morning, must wash out stool and backache; nauseous, bad taste in the morning, must wash out her mouth, produced by derangement of stomach; stools hard and large, after suppressed intermittent fever by quinine; alternate constipation and diarrhoea.
Ruta	Constipation following mechanical injuries; hard, scanty stool, frequent urging to stool, with protrustion of recutm when stooping ever so little and especially when squatting; copious flatus with the urging, constipation alternating with mucous, frothy stools.
Sanguinaria	Urging, but no stool, with sensation of a mass in lower part of rectum, and discharge only of offensive flatus; torpid liver, goneness in stomach, with sick headache.
Sanicula	(Mineral spring, Ills)—constipation, with ineffectual urging, no power to expel the stool, though straining with all his might and pressing until head feels as if it would burst; stool which seems to be at the verge of anus recedes, sometimes must be extracted with fingers.
Selenium	Atony of intestines; no peristaltic action; impaction of faeces which become hard and dry from absorption of the moisture and require artificial removal (Alum., Op., Plumb.); momentarily > from stimulants.

Continued...

Sepia	An all-gone feeling in rectum, inability to expel faeces or to strain at stool, with sensation of a ball in rectum; constipation of females, with pain and pressure in iliac regioins, from uterine or abdominal congestion; constipation during pregnancy; constant full feeling, as of a weight in rectum, even after a stool, with darting pains up rectum. Stool hard, knotty, difficult, a little of mucus-covered faeces is discharged off and on, but gives no satisfaction; prolapsus recti; soreness between buttocks; painfuil sensation of emptiness in pit of stomach; <from milk or fat pork; > to draw up limbs, when walking quickly, drinking cold water; hypochondriasis with aversion to family and to household duties.
Silicea	Stool of large, hard lumps, which remain long in rectum, and when after violent efforts of the abdominal muscles the faeces are nearly expelled, they as suddenly recede into the rectum, EVEN A SOFT STOOL IS EXPELLED WITH MUCH DIFFICULTY; soreness, stitches and shooting pains in anus or extreme hunger, hands and feet cold; constipation of women before and during menses, of scrofulous children.
Stannum	Costiveness in nursing women and in children, stools, though not very hard, are difficult to discharge from weakness of bowels; dry stools of round lumps, but of too large a size; discharge of a tough, hard part with straining; bitter or sour taste, yellow tongue. Pressure in stomach; loss of will and energy, restlessness or silent moroseness.
Staphisgria	Retarded stool on account of lack of peristaltic action, hard, scanty stool, with cutting and burning in anus; hard stool and flatus alternately; difficult stool with great distress, as if the rectum or anus were constricted, first with hard, then with soft faeces, or with only soft stool. Gouty person of a strumous diathesis, who lived too well for their own benefit. Colic with incarcertated flatus and gnawing, darting pains, > by passing flatus.

Strontia	Stools large and hard, expelled with great effort, followed by great pain in anus of a burning character, lasting for a long time, > by lying down; anus violently contracted after stool; coldness in spots on calves of legs.
Sulphur	Habitual constipation, especially in haemorrhoidal and hypochondriac people, complaining of dull feeling in brain, heaviness on top of head, weak, hungry sensation in stomach about noon, burning of the soles of feet at night; hard, insufficient, difficult stool, with fullness, heat and itching at anus, flat like sheep's dung, first effort so painful that patient stops straining; stool hard and black, as if burnt; constipation of infants; aversion to meat, sleep short and broken, frequent faint spells.
Tabacum	Desire for stool without any evacuation; after frequent but ineffectual attempts, a hard stool several hours after the regular time; habitual constipation, tympanitic abdomen, strangulated hernia, with nausea, deathly faintness, cold sweat.
Tarentula Cubana	Stools very dark, foetid, only partly formed, containing much mucus, expelled with difficulty and followed by burning and a smarting in anus; but no tenesmus. STOOL IMMEDIATELY ON HAVING THE HEAD WASHED.
Thuja	Obstinate constipation, inactivity of intessusception; hard, thick and knotty balls with pain in anus, when passing, as if it would fly to pieces, after stool repeated urging without accomplishing anything; smarting of anus between intervals of stools, OFFENSIVE PERSPIRTION AT ANUS AND PERINEUM; ineffectual desire for stool, accompanied by erections; constnt craving for salt.
Titanium	Obstinate constipation, no stool without injections; swelling and hardness of abdomen; pains in right side and back; foetid erucations and flatus; EXCREMENTS AT TIMES OF LITTLE BLACK PIECES LIKE GRAINS OF COFFEE.

Continued...

Veratrum Alb.	Constipation of infants; CHRONIC CONSTIPATION; INERTIA OF RECTUM (Op.), general depression of vitality; predominant coldness of the body; first portion of stool is large and the latter part consists of thin strings; stools very large and very hard; very weak after stool, or strains at stool until he is covered with cold sweat and then gives up exhausted, tired of life and afraid to die; craves cool and refreshing things.
Verbascum	Knoty stool like sheep's dung, passed after much effort; darting pains about navel, as if bowels adhered to the peritoneum and were being pulled out; sticking, constricting pains about navel; indurations.
Viburnum Opulus	Stools large, hard; dry balls, voided with much difficulty so as to need mechanical aid; much tenesmus during and after stool or inactivity of rectum; dark blood after stool; unable to concentrate mind on her usual labor.
Zincum	Dry, brittle, granular stool, which is passed only after prolonged effort, followed by involuntary micturition; violent bearing down in abdomen, <by passing flatus up and down; venous congestion in abdominal organs; hypochondriasis: < by wine.

A **Repertory** of the Constipation Remedies is given below: Repertory denotes the symptoms with the list of Remedies. Out of which the correct similimum should be selected. i.e. the remedy which cover all the symptoms of the ailment. Where there are more one symptom the remedy should all such symptoms. **It is suggested the remedy selected in each case should be referred from the list of Remedies given below the Repertory**

CONSTIPATION – Repertory – Remedies	
Symptoms	**Remedies**
Principal	Aesculus, Aletris., aloes, Baptisia, Bryonia, Calcarea carb., Carbo.veg., Chelidoniam, Collinsonia., dioscorea., Graphitis., Hydrastis., Iris Vers., Lycopodium., Natrum Mur., Nux.Vomica., Opium., Platinum., Plumbum., Podophylum., Pulsitilla., Sulphur., Veratrum alb.,
Habitual	Abies Nig., alumen., alumina., Bryonia., Calcarea., Causticum, Collinsonia., conium., Graphites,, Lachesis., Lycopodium., Sepia., Sulph., Fel turi or Fel vulp.
Persons who lead a sedentary life.	Aloes, Bryonia., Iris vers., Hydrastis., Lycopodium., Nux. vom., Opium., Platinum., Podophylum., Sulphur.
Abuseof Cathartics or after Diarrhoea/ Drunkards	Agaricus., Ant.crud. Bryonia, Lachesis., Nux.vom., Ruta. Agaricus; Lachesis.; Nux.vom; Opium; Sulphur.
Old People	Aloes., Alumina., Ant. Crud., Baryta Card., Bryonia., Lachesis., Opium., Phosphorus., Phytolacca., Rhus Tox., Ruta
Large eaters	Aloes, Dioscoria
Pregnant Women	Alumina Bryonia Lycopodium Nux.vom Opium Podophylum Sepia
-do – of lying-in wemen	Ant.crud., Ambra., Bryonia, Conium., Nux.vom Platinum
Constriction of Anus	Alumina, Bellodona, Causticum.,, Colchicum., Kali bich., Lycopodium Natrum Mur Nit.acid., Nux.vom Plumb.,,, Sepia., Silicea., Staph., Cocculus., Ignasia., Mezeriu., Srasparilla., Secale.,
Constriction after stool	Ignasia Colch., Kali bich, Nit.acid., Sepia, Sulphur

Continued...

When travelling	**Alumina; Magn.acet., Ignasia; Opium; Platinum.,**
From poisining of Lead	Aesculus; Opium; Platinum; Sulphur
Urine retained	Hyosimus
Ineffectual urging	1ˢᵗ – **grade**: Caps.; Conium; Lachesis; Lycopodium; Merc. Sol.; Nux.vom Sepia; Sulphur – 2ⁿᵈ **Grade**: Arnica; Bellodona; Calcarea carb; Carbo veg.; Causticum; Cocculus; Graphites; Ignatia; Kalmia; Natrum Mur; Nit.acid; Pulsitilla Silicea; Staph; Veratrum Alb; Zincum 3ʳᵈ **Grade**: *Aesculus hip.*; Ambra; Anacardium; Asaram; Hydrastis;. Phytolacca; Podophylum.
Without least desire as from inactivity of the bowels	1ˢᵗ – **grade** *Aethusa;* Alumina; China; Hepar sulf; Kalmia; Natrum Mur;*Nux.vom*; Staph; Thuja; Veratrum Alb 2ⁿᵈ **Grade**: Anacardium; Arnica; Bryonia; Carbo veg; Cocculus Graphites, Ignatia; Lycopodium; Magn. Mur; Natrum Mur; Nux.vom Opium; Petrolium; Rhododendran; Ruta; Sepia; Silicea; Sulphur – 3ʳᵈ **Grade**: Collins.; Gels.; Hydr.; Podo.
When faeces very hard	1ˢᵗ – **grade**: Alumen Amm.mur *Ant.* Mur.; *Ant. Crud.*; Bryonia; *Calcarea;* Carbo veg; Conium; Gauaiacum; *Lachesis;* Magn. Mur; Opium; *Plumbum; Sepia;* Silicea; *Sulphur:* 2ⁿᵈ **Grade** – Alumen Apis; Aur.Met; Carb.an.; Causticum.; Kalmia; *Lycopodium;* Magn. Carb; *Merc.; Nux vom*; Petrolium;. Rhus Tox; Ruta., Spong., Staph; Sulphur ac.; Thuja: 3ʳᵈ **Grade**: *Aesc.*hip; Fel tauri; Fel vulpis

When lumpy like sheep's dung	**1ˢᵗ – grade**: Alumen; Ignatia Merc.; Opium; Sepia; *Silicea*; Sulphur: **2ⁿᵈ Grade**: Amm.Mur; Baptisia; Baryta Carb;. Carb.an.; Causticum Graphites; Kalmia; *Lachesis*; Mangnam; Nux vom; Petrolium; Plumbum; Stannum; Sulphur ac.; Thuja; Veratrum Alb:
When too large	**1ˢᵗ – grade**: Ant.Crud.; Apis., *Bryonia*; *Calcarea*; Kalmia; Mgt.arc. Nux vom: **2ⁿᵈ Grade**: Aurum Met; Graphites; Ignatia; Magn. mur;Merc.; Stannum; Sulphur ac; Thuja; Veratrum Alb; Zincum:
When too thin	Causticum; *Graphites*; Hyoscimus; Merc.; *Mur.ac.*; Natr. Mur.; Puls. Sepia; Staphisgria:
When too scanty:	**1ˢᵗ – grade**: Alumen; Arnica; *Calcare;a* Graphites; Lycopodium Magn. Mur.; *Natr.Mur.*; Nux vom: Sepia; Silicea; *Sulphur* **2ⁿᵈ Grade**: Ars alb.; Bapisia; Baryta Carb.; Chamomilla;. China Lach., Ruta Stann. Staph. Zinc.
PROLAPSUS ANI – REMEDIES	
Arnica	Burning of hot spots on top of head; state of mind very pitiable; after a little walk the prolapsus protrudes and hinders him fromgoing any farther; during headache the rectum does not fall down and vice ersa.
Calcarea carb	Prolapsus ani during cholera infantum; burning with stool; itching; inflamed eruption around anus
Euphrasia	Prolapsus of ani from pressure in anal region when sitting; protrusion of large varices from anus
Ferrum	Prolapsus recti in children; itching in anus at night, from worms, protrusion of large varices at anus.
Hydrastis	Simple prolapsus in children with congestion and swelling of he mucous membrane and marked constipation.

Continued...

Ignatia	Prolapsus with or without piles. Sharp stabling pains shooting up into the the rectum; annoying patient, even if there is soft stool; constriction at anus; < after stool,> while sitting.
Lachesis	Prolapsis followed by painful constriction of anus; rectum prolapsed and tumefied; haemprrhoids protruding, with stitches upward when coughing or sneezing; sensation in rectum as if little hammers ere beating there.
Mercurias	Prolopsis ani with much straining, it looks dark and bloody; a sensation of "cannot-get-done feeling (Sulph), with beating
Muriatic acid	Prolapsus ani while urinating; piles in children, too sore to bear evev the least touch, protruding, bluish, burning.
Podophillum	Prolapsus ani before evacuation of faeces; anus extremely sore; sensation of weakness in abdomen and rectum, which remains protruding for a long time, especially in children.
Psorinum	Prolapsus recti, with burning and sticking, even asoft stool is voided with difficulty, from sheer weakness.
Ruta	Prolapsus from exhaution of muscular structure of bowels, as in children who are permitted to sit too long at stool or to strain too much or in adults after an attack of dysentery.

PROLAPSUS – INFANTUM – OF THE RECTUM

Prolapsus of the rectum is observed in **children**. In its management of the buttocks should be raised and the bowel carefully replaced. To assist in retaining it a strip of adhesive plaster about two inches wide should bind the buttocks together. This should be left in position when the bowels move, after which the parts should be thoroughly cleansed, and another piece applied. A remedy should be selected that will meet the totality of the condition.

PROLAPSUS – INFANTUM – REMEDIES	
Aloes	Should be studied in cases that are associated with diarrhea and dysentry and tenesmus, when the stools may be passed involuntarily, or when the desire for stool is imperative. Mercurious should be compared.
Calc. Carb.	Should be remembered in chronic cases in children
Ferr. Phos	Is frequently indicated in weakly, delicate, anemic children.
Ignatia	Is useful in nervous, hysterical subjects who are constipated. If the patient is a child it is fretful, cries and the anus is bluish and bloody and defecation is painful. The prolapsus appears from the least exertion.
Muriatic Acid	Should be studied in those cases in which the prolapsus occurs during micturition
Podophyllum	Should be studied in cases that occur following stool, muscular efforts, coughing, sneezing etc. the condition often has morning aggravation.
Sepia	Should be remembered in those cases that are made worse by any form of motion.

HEMORRHOIDS

Aetiology: They are most common in middle life. They may be dependent upon a local pressure which interferes with the current of blood as constipation, tumors of the rectum, enlargement of the uterus and ovaries, enlarged prostate, strictures of the rectum, especially as a result from syphilis. Interference with the portal circulation, as is found in hepatic atrophic cirrhosis and hepatic congestion, and diseases of the heart and lungs that interfere with the return of blood by the general venous circulation are also causes of haemorrhoids. An excess of food and a lack of exercise predispose hemorrhoids. They are common in gouty, obese subjects, and in men more frequently than in women.

Pathology: Hemorrhoids may be situated above or below the sphincter ani. If above they are known as internal haemorrhoids, while below the sphincter are known as external. They may appear as irregular links surrounding the anus, and are of a bluish colour, and vary in size. Internal haemorrhoids are usually broad and flat and at times pedunculated and may protrude through the sphincter ani. Inflammation of the surrounding mucous membrane is usually present. The haemorrhoids may undergo ulceration and suppuration, hemorrhage may occur, thrombosis may be formed in the veins and fistula develop.

Symptoms: Auxilliary treatment: These vary according to the extent of the process. Frequently they cause great annoyance; there is pain of a burning, smarting character and sensation in the rectum as if it were filled with foreign body. The pain is aggravated during defecation, by long continued sitting and by horseback riding. Nausea, vomiting and palpitation of the heart may accompany these symptoms. Internal haemorrhoids produce a sensation of fullness in the rectum and a dull aching pain and frequently a muco-purulent bloody discharge. The hemorrhage may be profuse. When the haemorrhoids prolapsed and become strangulated the pain is intense. People should ensure regular evacuation of the bowels. Alchoholic and sexual excesses should be avoided. If the haemorrhoids are inflamed and protruding the patient should remain in bed, and a soothing application should be applied, as warmed witch-hazel or calendula, or a cerate prepared from these. I they fail to bring relief, a poultice of flax-seed or cornmeal and onions should be applied, and changed from time to time to keep it warm. In some cases the holding of a piece of ice to the part or spraying with cold water has relieved the engorgement. If the hemorrhage is severe whenever the bowels move, it will be found that a teaspoonful of **Hamamelis** in a half glass of water taken internal three times a day for a month, then twice a day for month, then once a day for another month will correct the condition.

HEMORRHOIDS REMEDIES	
Aesculus Hip	Is an important remedy in many of these cases. The haemorrhoids may be either internal or external. They are hard, purple, very tender, ache and burn. The patient complains of a sensation of dryness, soreness, constriction and fullness or as if ticks, gravel or splinters were lodged in the rectum. The sensation of fullness and protrusion is associated with that of tenesmus and a desire to strain. There is a severe backache with lameness, aching and weakness which is referred to the back.
Aloes	Is indicated when the haemorrhoids protrude like bunches of grapes. There is a const ant bearing down sensation. The discharge of blood is black. There is a degree of tenderness and congestion of the liver. The distress caused by the haemorrhoids is relieved by the application of cold.
Collinsonia	Is useful in the cases in which constipation is a prominent factor. The constipation is obstinate and habitual. The stools are lumpy and light coloured
Hamamelis	Should be studied in cases when there are varicose veins. The haemorrhoids bleed profusely. The blood is venous; there is itching, burning and rawness of the anus.
Nux Vom.	Should be remembered in those of sedentary habits who indulge in liquors and highly seasoned food. The bowels are constipated and there is more or less abdominal distress. In most of the cases, Sulphur 30 at 8 a.m. and Nux vom 30 at 4 p.m. for about 3 to 4 days gives relief – or start the treatment as above in each case and when relief I not there the next indicated remedy could be studied.
Sulphur	Is indicated in persons who are subject to venous congestion, especially of the portal system. They are subject to alternate constipation and diarrhea. The stools are blood streaked. There is frequently protruding of the piles which bleed and there is a sensation of burning and itching after the stool as well as tenesumus
Also study Aconite, Capscicum, Ars. Alb. And Podophyllum	

FISSURES OF THE ANUS

Symptoms:

A vertical tear of lining of anus, a painful condition with anal sphincter in spasm. The principal symptom is the paroxysm of pain which accompanies defecation; as if a red hot iron were boring through the anus. The pain may extend to the genital organs, legs, and bladder. On account of the severe pain, the patient defers defecatioin or even passing of flatus. Inspection and digital examination real the fissure, at the external end of which there is a polypoid fold of the skin.

FISSURES OF THE ANUS – (Fissura-ano) Remedies	
Aesculus hip:	Anus feels raw, soreness, burning, itching and fullness at anus;' pain like a knife sawing backward and forward through anus; pain in anus about an hour after stool, continuing for some time.
Berberies vul.	Great soreness and pain throughout entire back, from sacrum to shoulders, < by any physical labour; dry, troublesome cough; acrid leucorrhoeal discharge, very prostrating in its effects; violent burning pains in anus during stool, as if surrounding parts were sore, frequent and constant desire to stool.
Causticum	Fissures which tend to dry up and have dark-brown or purple edges; walking causes pain in bleeding from anus.
Graphites	Fissures of recent origin, especially in children; varices of rectum and burning rhagades between them. Fissures caused by large faecal masses, no irritability, no frequent desire to stool nor spasmodic contraction of sphincter, only some smarting and soreness, < at night and when sitting; flatus rancid or putrid.
Hydrastis	Burning and smarting pain in rectum and anus after each stool, lasting for hours, with hot sensation in bowels, colic and faintness, stools dry, large, lumpy, nodulated; dyspeptic cough with espectoration of ropy mucous.

Ignatia	Fissures with haemorrhoids and polapsus recti, with pains shooting upward in the rectum after stool, particularly a loose stool; pains return at the same hour each day,< from walking or standing.
Lachesis	Sensation of little hammers pecking away in fissured parts; tormenting urging, but not to stool; itching at anus, < after sleep.
Nitric acid	Sharp, splinter-like cutting pains in rectum during and burning after stool; painful prolapsus of bowels and sensation of constriction in anus; very irritable, thinks will never be improving.
FISSURES OF THE ANUS – (Fissura-ano) Remedies	
Paeonia	Ulcerations of mucous membranes of rectum and anus, with fissures burning and biting some hours after stool; parts swollen and exhaling an offensive odour; diarrhoea with colic; anus damp and disagreeable from constant oozing.
Platina	Fissura ani with crawling and itching in anus every evening; frequent urging with scanty stool; painful sensation of weaknes
Rhatanhia	Burning in the anus like fire, preceding and accompanying defecation and lasting long time after, accompanied by prostration of varices; dry heat anus, with sudden stitches like stabs with pen – knife; sensation as if the rectum protruded and went back with a jerk, with most horrible pains; frequent and ineffectual desire to urinate; burning in urethra while urinating.
Rhus Tox	Fissura ani with periodical bleeding from anus; blind piles protruding after stool, with pressure in rectum as if everything would come out.
Sepia	Constructive pain in rectum, extending to perineum and into the vagina; pain in rectum on going to stool, which persists for a long time after sitting down.

Continued...

Silicea	Long and painful efforts to expel the contents of the rectum but the sphincter ani seems tightly to resist the effort till suddenly the stool passes, sometimes with pain and nervous shuddering; stool partly descends and then slips back again.
Sulphuric acid	Sensation as of rectum being torn as under during defaecation, lancinating pains running upward from anus.
Thuja	Fissures with edges trimmed with polypoid excrescenes or true rectal polypus; piles, condylomata, urinary troubles.

FISTULA ANUS

(Fistula – ano)

Anterior fistula communicates directly with anal canal and posterior fistula is always horse-shoe in type entering the anal canal in the mid line:

Aloe, Aurum mur. Berberies vul., Ignatia, Kreosote, Lachesis, Nux. vom., Sepia, Silicea, Staphisgria, Sulphur.—**Helmuth** recommends Merc.sol. Hep., Hep Sil. To hasten the breaking of the abcess, and Phosphorouswhere there is complication with pulmonary affections. The dyspepsia may require Calc. Merc.sol. Nux.Vom. Silicea, Sulph.

Fistula Anus: – Remedies	
Aloe	Heaviness and stricture of rectum; sensatgion of heat and burningin rectum; itching, pulsating in rectum < sitting; after stool burning weight and itching in anus; cutting as if till more would come; fullness and pressing out of the anus.
Berberies vul.	Violent burning in anus, as if surrounding parts were sore; frequent and constant desire for stool, burning stitching pains during before and after into (left side of) pelvis; tearing extending around anus; short cough and chest complaints; biliary colic; tetter on edge of anus.

Calc. Phos.	After surgical interference for the fistula. FISTULA ANI ALTERNATING WITH CHEST SYSTEMS or in persons who have pains in joints with every spell of cold stormy weather, especially in tall, sore feeling in anus when getting up in the morning.
Causticum	Frequent, sudden, penetrating, pressive pain in rectum; anus very sensitive to contact; itching and stickling in rectum.
Hydrdastis	Fistula ani with constipation, piles and ulceration; offensive, dirty – looking discharge from anus, obliging him to wear a bandage.
Lachesis	Fistula in drunkards, with discharge to pulmonary complications
Nux. Vom.	Gastrosis and constipation, < after mental exertions, after eating.
Silicea	FISTULA IN ANO WITH CHEST SYMPTOMS: sharp stitches in rectum while walking; abdominal pains> by warmth; suppuration of abscess; purulent sputa.

CHAPTER – 9

PEPTIC ULCERS & TREATMENT

A KALEIDOSCOPIC VIEW & AETIOLOGY OF PEPTIC ULCER

In Greek the word 'Pepsis' relates to "Digestion" and the term Pepsein" conveys the meaning as "to Digest". The word "Peptic", however, concerns regarding "Digestion" and Pepsin" and the ulcer or sore joins with this and thus we get the name of a disease" Peptic Ulcer" which is becoming one of the major diseases of the modern world.

Peptic Ulcer is a broad term used generally for denoting an ulcer or sore that either occurs in the lower end of the esophagus, along the lesser curvature of stomach, in the duodenum or on jejunal side of the gatro-jejunestomy, deriving commonly the name as gastric ulcer or duodenal ulcer, accordingly.

Aetiologically speaking, there are many factors existing for this disease like the predisposing, **Acid**, traumatic, vascular, toxic, neurogenic, **vitamin deficiency**, **diet factors** etc. but, as both "psyche" the mind and "soma" the body take part along with other factors in establishing this disease, it is generally to be grouped, into the "psychosomatic" diseases'.

Accordingly to one authority it is estimated that peptic ulcer is a condition which is said to occur one time or another in 10% of the population. Peptic ulcer of chronic type is more common in men than in women. The proportion of chronic ulcers today occurring in the duodenum is, however, 80% and needless to say that it has become now-a-days a major problem, when our eyes embrace the printed letter of the news, often, about suicide of such victims due to intolerance of its pain or so.

Allopathically speaking, according to Dr. Fenwick, it comes probably as a small abasing crack or fissure, which deepens quickly and may thereby involve an arteriole and cause bleeding preceded by pain, and vomiting. The progress is sometimes so rapid that perforation occurs, owing to the lack of defensive reaction in the peritoneum. It is probably due to largely an infective condition of the mouth and teeth or sometimes of the appendix of biliary passages. The gastric juice secreted by the mucous membranes of the stomach is approximately five million gallons during average life span and is clear colourless acid fluid of a low specific gravity containing over 90% water, the remainder is partly organic and partly inorganic matter in solution. It contains 0.7% of free hydrochloric acid, which is very powerful to cut into pieces the food it acts upon. The walls of the stomach would ordinarily beat away by this strong acid but for the fact that they are continually protected by alkaline secretion by the mucous membranes of the stomach.

Pathology of Gastric Ulcer:

Acute ulcer is small and presents an appearance of having been punched out of the mucous membrane. Chronic ulcer is funnel shaped, its apex extending towards the peritonea cover, while its edges are thickened owing to an increase of the fibrous tissue of the stomach. Adhesions may be found between the stomach and surrounding organs. Acute ulcers occur most frequently about the pyloric orifice and the first part of the duodenum, 40 per cent being upon the posterior (back) surface of the stomach, 26 per cent upon the lesser curvature, 15 per cent at the pyloric orifice, 6 per cent, on the anterior (front) surface, 11 per cent in the greater curvature and a 2 per cent at the cardiac orifice.

The ulcer may cicatrise or perforate. When cicatrisation takes place, hour glass contraction of stomach may result, but in other cases when the ulcer is situated near the pyloric or the esophageal orifice a stenosis (narrowing) may form. Perforation occurs as a result of muscular effort or by an acute ulcerative process. It frequently accompanies those ulcers that occur upon the anterior and posterior surface and on the lesser curvatures.

Gastric ulcers occur as a result of injury to the tissues, the invasion of bacteria and some interference with the circulation of blood to the part. Chronic ulcers are frequently due thrombosis dependent upon gastric juices. The secretion of gastric juice may be normal or it may be increased and hyperchlorhydia may be present. In cases of pulmonary tuberculosis complicated with gastric ulcer there is often a diminished acidity of the stomach. Gastric myasthenia, muscular irritability that results in spasm, gastric dilation, and hour glass contraction may result.

Pathological symptoms.:

Cellular infiltration, fibrosis, erosion, superficial erosion of gastric mucosa, haemorrhage, haematemesis, i.e vomiting food.

Latest theory for formation of Peptic Ulcers – pathological symptoms:

H pyloric infection, appears to be main cause of Gastritis or Peptic Ulcers. H pylori is a spiral gram negative rod that resides beneath the gastric mucous layer adjacent to gastric epithelial cells. Although it is not invasive, it causes gastric mucosal inflammation with poly morph nuclear netrophills and lymphocytes. The **pathology** of injury and inflammation in part may be related to the products of two genes, vacA and cagA.

Acute infection with H pylori may cause a transient clinical illness characterized by nausea and abdominal pain that may last for several days and is associated with acute histological gastritis with poly morphonuclear neutrophills and lymphocytes. Inflammation may be confined to the superficial gastric epithelium or may extend deeper into the gastric glands resulting in varying degrees of gland atrophy (atrophic gastritis) and metaplasia of the gastric epithelium to intestinal type epithelium. H pylori infection is also responsible for formation of peptic ulcer due to such chronic inflammation in the mucous quotes of stomach or duodenum as the case may be.

SYMPTOMS AND SIGNS

Epigastric pain (dyspepsia) the hall mark peptic ulcer disease, is present in **80–90%** of patients. However, this complaint is not sensitive or specific enough to serve as a reliable diagnostic criterion for peptic ulcer disease. The clinical history cannot accurately distinguish duodenal from gastric ulcers. **Less than one-quarter of patients with** *dyspepsia* have ulcer disease at endoscopy. Upto 20% of patients with ulcer complications such as bleeding have no antecedent symptoms (silent ulcers).

Pain is typically well **localized** to the **epigastrium** and not severe. It is described as gnawing, dull, acting, or "hunger-like". Classic features of peptic ulcer pain is rhythimicity and periodicity. Rhythimicity means that the pain fluctuates in intensity through out the day and night. Approximately half of patients get relief of cause nocturnal pain that awakens the patient. A change from a patient's typical rhythmic discomfort to constant or radiating pain may reflect ulcer penetration or perforation. Most patients have symptomatic periods lasting upto several weeks patients.

Pain in Gastric ulcer may come immediately after taking food. Pain is dull, continuous ache, or deep burning in character more often occurring in a rhythmic manner. It may reappear every time on taking food or water, milk. At times pain is relieved after taking either solid or liquid food.

In Gastric ulcer the pain is mainly in the anterior aspect and immediately afterfood. In the duodenal ulcer the pain comes after two to four hours and extend to back as well as anterior aspect, when it is situated on the posterior part of the stomach. It may erode nearby viscera such as pancreas. In duodenal ulcer the pain may be there when stomach empty and there may be relief after taking something. **Periodicity of Pain:** *For about 15 days to 3 months the patient may suffer from the pain and it will subside for 23 months and reappear again. The revision is the very characteristic of peptic ulcer.*

FACTORS FOR FORMATION OF PEPTIC ULCERS AND SYMPTOMS

i) Continental theory for formation of peptic ulcer:

The formation of the Peptic ulcer is in considerable variation from place to place, time to time and also by climates, race and population. Sufferers from peptic ulcer are more in civilized society than the uncivilized society. For example, in Africa, the sufferers from peptic ulcer are more of white people than the local (native) black people. Many Doctors are suffering from peptic ulcer. Males preponderant than females. Most of the studies about peptic ulcer found that the ratio of Duodenal and Gastric ulcer is 18:1 respectively.

ii) Age group:

In males the age group between 30 to 50 years are prone to get peptic ulcer. Females during the age group between 30 to 45 years, are not prone to develop peptic ulcers, especially during child bearing period (during pregnancy). It is believed that there is some connection between female hormones and peptic ulcer. It is also believed that female hormone can help for not developing peptic ulcer. Before puberty and after menopause, the females also are prone to peptic ulcer.

iii) Hereditary factors:

It is not proved that the hereditary factors are responsible for formation of peptic ulcer.

iv) Food habits:

The persons who are in habit of taking spicy food are prone to get peptic ulcers.

(v) Blood Type – 'O' – Group:

Blood Type O may be predisposed to ulcers due to higher levels of stomach acid. The unique characteristic of type 'O' possess very well-developed ability to digest meals that contain both protein and fat.

These very same strengths come at a cost – in Type 'O' towards simple carbohydrates, especially from grains, are more *easily* converted into fats and triglycerides. Many grains also contain reactive proteins called lectins that can ramp up the type 'O' immune system, resulting in *unwanted inflammation* due to higher levels of stomach acid and auto-immunity. As such Dr. D'Adamo recommends following the type 'O' diet, which focuses on lean, organic meats, vegetable and fruits and avoid wheat and dairy which can be triggers for digestive and health issues in Type O.

Dr. D'Adamo suggests that type 'O's should avoid *caffeine and alcohol*. Caffeine cane be particularly harmful because of its to raise adrenaline and nonadrenaline, which are already high for type O's. and also to avoid sweets since produce hydrochloric acids in the digestive tract.

REASONS FOR PAIN IN THE PEPTIC ULCER

i) Presence of Hydrochloric acid:

It is found that one of the causes of pain in gastric ulcer and duodena ulcer is mainly due to hydrochloric acid in the stomach. A gastro-enterologist has done extensive work on this subject. He withdrew hydrochloric acid and injected hydrochloric after neutralizing the same. So he found out that the acid is the main cause of the pain.

ii) Motility theory:

This theory explains that the pain is caused by the spasm of gastric muscles or duodenal muscles (due to tension of egastric ulcers

iii) Inflammation theory:

Pain in the gastric or duodenal ulcer may be of any type. By the muscular contraction more the acid comes into contact with the surface of the narrow surroundings which is the cause for the production of the pain in peptic ulcer.

iv) Pain in peptic ulcer is in the posterior aspect dull, continuous deep ache, and radiating to back.

Diet to be avoided which has more acid:

- Beef, Bread white, Eggs, Oat meal, Oysters, Rice, Wheat whole, Cigar, Coffee, Condiments etc. Relief of the pain is found after ingestion of alkalies/Diet suggested containing Alkali
- Apples, Bananas, Cantaloupe, Carrots, Kale, Milk, Oranges, Pears, Potatoes, Tomatoes, Water, Melon.

PEPTIC ULCERS (TREATMENT)

In Homoeopathy, the fundamental principal is to **treat the patient as a whole.** Nevertheless, in clinical experience, it has been found that certain remedies found to act in a specific manner on peptic ulcers in different cases, and few of them may also be called *'pathological prescriptions'* and not individualistic. No doubt, this aspect also should be taken into consideration. We lay more stress on the *'psychic'* aspect not only for the causation, but also for the evolution and termination of diseases. Hence, the modern stresses and strains, late hours worries etc. predispose for such ulcer and if we enquire into these aspects while taking the case and prescribe for the preclinical stages, we will be able to nip the complaint in its bud. This first stage is the pre-ulcer stage, when the person looks healthy, having the above background of predisposing and exciting factors, established ulcer cases requires a patient and prolonged drug therapy, diet restriction and change in the mode of living and shaping the mental well being.

PEPTIC ULCERS: (remedies)	
Ars. Alb	Gastric Ulcer in stomach region or duodenal ulcer involving pancreas – Burning like vapour or hot water poured on the painful part of the stomach – > by hot drinks – ice water < – When peptic ulcer is at pyloric end – Duodinitis – or when Duodenal ulcer involves Pancreas – epigastric pain immediately after taking meals – The patient complains of great anxiety and gnawing pain that burns like fire in the stomach, which is sensitive to pressure – Neither food nor drink is retained in the stomach, and drinking is followed immediately by vomiting. Stomach tender to pressure, even to the slightest touch, gnawing in pit of stomach; vomiting of blood, with fainting before and after it; frequent vomiting; with apprehension of death; pain in stomach while or immediately after eating or gnawing, nausea and vomiting, mostly after two hours even from the lightest kind of food
Arg. Nit	Ulcer at the cardiac orifice of stomach with flatulency –pain in left side elbow, short ribs, and pain localised just below the xiphoid cartilage in a small spot, extending to a corresponding point in spine < by pressure – spasm across lower part of chest and in stomach due to ulceration in mucous membrane of stomach and duodenum coming on late evenings and lasting all night. The pain also radiates from the epigastrium to the shoulder, chest and abdomen. There is usually fermentation, and an examination of the blood shows a condition of chlorosis to be present. Craving for sweets but they aggravate.

PEPTIC ULCERS: (remedies)	
Anacardium	Gastric and duodenal ulcers < after 2 hours of eating – two will minded – indecisive plug feelings at different parts of the body – specific remedy for **duodenal ulcer** where the pain is there after two hours of eating < when the stomach is empty.
Adrenal cortex	When the indicated remedy does not work try "Adrenal Cortex"(Cortisone) in case of duodenal ulcer – it is found in provings that Adrenal cortex (Cortisone) produces Peptic Ulcer (Duodenal Ulcer)
Alum. Phos	Peptic ulcer of bleeding type
Bismuth Nit.	Sensation of pressure as from a load in one spot, and a pressing burning sensation extending from stomach through to the spine > by bending backward. There is continuous nausea and vomiting which relieved by cold drinks for a time, but the stomach becomes filed with fluid and vomited immediately
Condurango 6	Ulcer at **cardiac end of stomach or lower end of esophagus** – constant burning pain in stomach with no relation of food intake.
Carbo-veg.	Pain as if coals are burning with distension of abdomen > after ejection of gas – Burning below short ribs – dry mouth without thirst – **Acid dyspepsia** – Dyspepsia after loss of animal fluids i.e. blood, semen or sexual excesses and masturbation or sexual abuse – History of varicose veins – Pain extends backwards
Hydrastis	Great soreness and burning pain referred to the stomach. complains of a sensation of faintness and gone-ness in the epigastrium, **with hyperacidity** and nausea, vomiting and empty eructation. There are evidences of a catarrhal condition of the stomach with jaundice and torpidity of the liver.
Iodine	When there is relief of pain after cold milk in peptic ulcer try this remedy.

Continued...

Merc. Corr	When the epigastric region is distended and is extremely sensitive to the slightest pressure and there are sharp darting pains through it – Sore burning pain in the transverse colon
Ornithogalam Q	Gastric and Duodenal Ulcers – **Single drop Dose of mother tincture in half ounce water and observe.**
Robinia 6	Where the ulcer is due to **Hyper-acidity** and centred round about the intense acidity of the eructations
Symphytum	Peptic ulcer with history of sexual excesses
Uranium Nit	Gastric ulcer in diabetic patient/constant urging for urination – impotence –power of curing ulceration of the **pyloric end of the stomach and the upper portion of the duodenum**, indicated in the patient/great despondency and is ill-tempe. There are **burning pains in the pyloric region**, with intermittent attacks of pain in the epigastric region with acid eructations. Recurrent haematemesis. Vomiting of blood, tasteless or putrid eructations, great thirst, no appetite, styes on left upper eyelid; constipation, extreme debility and vomiting of white fluid.

PEPTIC ULCERS: Keep the following remedies in view	
Atropinum	Pressing pain after eating and vomiting of acrid, sour masses, which set on edge, hard swelling of pyloric region, just above the navel, very sensitive to touch, severe gastralgia, constant vomiting, deathly paleness of face, with cold perspiration, hands and feet icy cold, pulse very small; peritonitis from perforation (Bellodonna) – Frightful pain at cardiac end of stomach.
Cantharis	When there is violent burning in stomach, chiefly pyloric region; pressure in scrobiculum after eating ; vomiting water drunk, also of blood, or frothy mucus, tinged bright – red; thirst with aversion to all food, with urinary symptoms.
Graphites 6	With persisting scarring – Use for a week or a fortnight – Pain relieved after taking food and lying down – Persistant scarring with ulcer > after eating and lying down.

Hamamalis	Haemorrhage , blood black, violent throbbing or trembling of stomach; and sore abdomen.
Kali-Bich	< Immediately after eating – spot ulcers – spot pains – stringy mucus – rheumatic symptoms alternate gastric symptoms – Duodinitis (Inflammation of duodenum) Ulcer at cardiac end of Stomach– There is acidity of the stomach, with a sensation of pressure and burning, vomiting of bile, and of pinkish, glairy, tenacious fluid. The sensation of pressure and burning is aggravated after food – Oval Ulcers evacuavating in depth without spreading in circumference; pressure and heaviness in stomach after eating, dizziness followed by violent vomiting of a white mucus, acrid fluid, vomiting of sour, undigested food; of bile, with pinkish glairy fluid of blood, with cold sweat on hands, hot face
Lycopodium	Earthly colour of face; rising of sour, acrid fluid, vomiting of sour water and mucus; fullness of stomach and abdomen; cobnstipation; scanty Urine < from sitting bent > from rising and walking about, no pain at night in warm bed.
Mezereum	Constant violent pain and pressure in stomach after eating, even the simplest food, constrictive, squeezing pain, with much belching, one to two hours after eating – ending with vomiting, and gulping up of food; constipation; circumscribed redness of face; skin cool, pulse very small & frequent; chilliness, attending with flushes of heat.
Phosphorous	Burning pain relieved after drinking ice water till it becomes warm in the stomach – duodinitis – Sensation of burning heat in the extending to the back, and a faint empty feeling referred to the stomach and bowels. The extremities are cold, and there is vomiting after taking food, and of water that has taken a few minutes before minutes before.
Podophylum 1M & CM	Duodinitis – Obstruction due to Peptic Ulcer

Sensations	Remedy
Sensitiveness to pressure	Ars.Alb., Bell., Bryonia, Kali-bich., Phos
With diminished sensibility	Arg.Nit. Bismuth, Crb.Veg., Phos. Acid
Excessive Acidity	Calc.Carb., Nux-Vom., Phos., Sulph.
Loss of Appetite	Ars.Alb., Nux-vom
Bulimy	Calc.Carb., Calcarea iod., Nux.Vom., Phos.
Fainting	Ars.Alb., Phos., Veratrum Alb.
At pyloric end	Ars.Alb
At cardiac end of Stomach	Kali-bich., Phos.

CASES OF PEPTIC ULCERS TREATED

BY Dr. P. Sankaran

Case – 1:

Mr. G aged 39 years, turned up for consultation on 8th Nov. 1957 for the following complaints.

Attacks of flatulent colic > Flatus > fomentation, < potatoes, Onions, fruits especially Bananas and Coconut, rice & heavy food.

Sweats with abdominal pain – formerly abdominal pain > eating – Milk does not agree, causes diarrhoea, Cannot stand hunger – Prefers hot drinks – Lumbar ache < rising in morning > Pressure – previous history and family: Nil, Operated for right sided hydrocele, Wt. 120 lbs.

On Bariam Meal X-ray it showed an ulcer niche in duodenum with pseudo diverticuli due to adhesions – The radiologist considered that it must be a **chronic ulcer** – On reperterisation (Kent's Repertory) of the case it has come out as under:

Fruit + (p.1362) Onions <(p.1363) Lyco. – Puls.

+ Milk < (p.1362) Lyco. – Puls

+ Perspiration with pains (p.1299) Lyco.

Besides this Lyco also covered "Back pain" in Lumbar region, in the morning after rising from bed" and also the desire for hot drinks.

Lyco 10M three doses in one day and was put on bland diet – Response was very satisfactory.

On 24th Nov 1957 he reported that he had no pains, and no weakness. On 28th Feb. 1958 he reported that he had switched over to his regular diet of spicy food – for a fortnight and he was not getting pain. He had severe pain in abdomen and back.

Again he was put on a bland diet and was given three doses of Lyco 10M, all to be taken in one day. On 10th March 1958 he reported that he was on bland diet, but still he had discomfort and gas – slight pain < till digestion is finished. Wt.128 Lbs.

He was given three doses of Carbo Veg 10M because Carbo Veg is known to help and augment the action of Lyco. But in spite of this, on 14th March 1958 he reported that he had severe pain in abdomen extending to chest and back. Pain > rubbing, flatus, heat and eructations. I now gave him three doses of Lyco 10M.

On 12th April 1958 he reported that he had slight pain and was on bland diet, no gas trouble – wt. 124 lbs. Again Lyco 10M three doses were given.

On 28th April 1958, he reported that his condition was much better and that there was no pain. He had started taking his regular diet. Barium meal X ray now showed Ulcer healing but still very deep. The radiologist felt that it was a case for surgery. On 2nd July 1960 the patient reported that he had been free from pain for last one and half, years, though on normal diet. He had to take only occasional doses of Lyco 10M. Now one dose of Lyco 50M is given. In 1964 he sent me a report that he was completely well for the last four years without any medicine and on normal diet. He also sent me another patient of peptic ulcer.

Case – 2:

Mr. PS aged 24 years consulted me on 21st Oct. 1954 for te following complaints.

Past two months no appetite – Distension after eating flatus and eructatiions give relief – Stitching pain abdomen, especially on right side, travelling to chest and back.

Takes food at 8.30 a.m. pain starts after 11.30 am and stops at once on taking any food or drink – hot or cold – stops for an hour or two and reappears after 3 p.m. but then it is not much relieved by food or drink. It continues till 9 p.m. till he takes his dinner and thereafter it subsides. Eructations all the twenty four ours – Gets frequent colds – Dislikes cold drinks, sweets. Thirst 8 to 10 glasses per day – Feels weak – Memory poor – especially now-a-days – smokes heavily.

At a leading hospital in Bombay all investigations had been done and it had been diagnosed as gastric ulcer – The following were taken into consideration and the case was repertorised as follows on Phatak's Repertory –

< Long after eating (P.77) + Eating >amel (p.77) – Anac. Kali-Bich

+ direction Ascending (p.67) – Kali Bich

+ Directon Backward (p.67) – Kali Bich

He was given three doses of Kali Bich. 200 in one day.

Then I did not see him to the next two years and nine months but thereafter he reported that he had no pains at all after taking the doses of Kali Bich. He had been completely normal. **Now he had merely come to thank me and to introduce one more patient. I hear in 1966 he still remains well.**

Case – 3:

Mr. P – aged 30 years came to me for consultation on 8th Oct 1956 with the following complaints:

Last year in June he had recurrent pain in abdomen which lasted for three months. He became free in Sept. but two months back i.e. in August this year he had a relapse. He now has epigastric pain which starts at 7 a.m. remains for fifteen minutes and then recurs at 11 or 11.30 a.m. remains for thirty minutes and again starts at 3 p.m. lasting for two hours and comes back at 1 am. Lasting for half an hour. The pain wakes him up from sleep at night. The pain usually starts two or three hours after food except at night when it occurs four hours after food. This pain > eating anything, soda lemon, salt. **If he is on milk diet he has no pain.** Appetite normal: Likes warm tea, food etc. Thirst: five glasses per day likes cold water. Stools are irregular: Sleep – good sweat – normal: Likes open air – Get headache by sitting under the fan wt. 119 lbs.

He was admitted to the govt. Homoeopathic Hospital and an X ray was taken, showed: **'Duodenal Ulcer'**

The following symptoms were taken and the case was repertised as under following **Boger's Synoptic key:**

Pain > eating (p.77) + Pain< long after eating (p.77) – Anac., Kali Bich., Nat Mur: Phos.

He was then given Anacardium 200 with no result. So his **case taken again** and this revealed one more symptom viz. that he also gets wandering pains in the abdomen which is in spots and which last for only two or three minutes – Now on the basis of this additional information, **Kali Bich** was selected. On 22nd Oct he was given three doses of **Kali Bich 30** – He had immediate relief and on 1st Nov 196 he reported that even though he takes spicy food sometimes, there is no pain – He took no more medicine and ten years later on 24th March 1966, **he reported that he has remain well all these years.**

Case – 4:

Sri KSM aged 39 years, came to me for consultation on 5th July 1963 with the following history:

In June 1946 he had an attack of **haemophysis**. It was suspected as food poisoning and treated as such. Five months later he had pain in the abdomen. X-ray was taken and the case was diagnosed as **duodenal ulcer** *with amoebic infection superadded*. He took some allopathic medicines. Since then he has pain on and off. Once again an X-ray was taken on 17th March 1963 after he had an attack of severe vomiting and dehydration. The X-ray showed **"old duodenal ulcer and spasm"**. Now he gets abdominal distension 2 to 3 hours after food with **burning eructations which gives some relief. Eructations Vomiting also gives some relief.** The vomitus is extremely sour. He does not get any trouble on empty stomach. He has constipation: has frequent urging with scanty stool. He has to strain even for a soft stool. He feels suffocated in closed room. He prefers to sleep on the cold floor. He has flatulence on right side. He feels > lying on left side < lying on back and right side. Thirst – takes only one cone cup of water day. Now-a-days he does not perspire but feels > if he perspires. If he sleeps in the afternoon, vomits on getting up. He feels suffocated in closed room. He prefers to be alone. He is very nervous and irritable but suppresses anger and brood, is oversensitive and very punctual in his work.

(Aetiology i.e. route cause) Past history: He had smallpox at the age of six months. He got disappointed in Oct. 1945 because he was not allowed to appear in a departmental examination. He has grief due to loss of son aged 2 in 1951, **but he suppressed his grief**. On examination, BP 110/80. His weight which was originally 120 lbs is now 101 lbs.

The case was repertorised as follows in Kent's repertory.

Lying on back < (p.1372) + Lying on right side < (p.1373): Acon., Alum., Am.carb., amm.mur., bor., bufo.,caust., merc., phos., ran.bulb., spong., sul., thuj.

Perspiration, suppressed complaints: Acon., Bry., Merc., Nux-v., Phos., Sulphur from (p.1302):

+Constipation, difficult stool (p.607): Bry, Merc., Nux-v. Phos., Sulph

+Grief ailments from (p.51): Nux.V:

+ Brooding (p.10) Nux. V.

+Eructations, foul: (p.495) Nux.V

Nux.Vom., covered many other symptoms of the patient, and seemed to match the totality – So I gave on 19–7-63 Nux.Vom 200 three doses a day for 3 days.

22–07–63: Patient feels weak, Flatus + + Pain same.,: **Nux-Vom 1M** twice a day for four days

30–7-63: Patient feels **much better** – Nux.Vom 1M daily once for seven days

05–8-63: Pain nil: **Feels > Nux.vom., 1 M** daily once for seven days

14-8-63: Patient **feels > Flatus > Nux.Vom., 10M** three doses in one day followed by placebo (i.e. sugar pills)

30-8-63: Patient had vomiting on 25th with pain: otherwise much better Nux Vom 10 M three doses in one day followed by placebo. **Three years later I heard that the patient remains well.** Unfortunately follow up X-ray could not be taken.

Case – 5:

Mr. SSB aged 46 years came to me for consultation on 17th April 1963 with the following history:

Patient suffering from duodenal ulcer since 1956. Originally it had been diagnosed as hyper-acidity but later X-ray revealed the lesion. Pain in abdomen is relieved by taking food or milk.

The pain at once > by passing flatus, >stretching < by pressure < wearing light clothes around the abdomen.

He has constipation and piles and has to strain even for soft stool. Milk and rice cause flatulence. He smokes 30 cigaretes a day for last 20 years. He is outwardly calm and unperturbed but actually he suppresses his feelings. He keeps things to himself. In past history he had suffered from malaria. In 1961 he also had a shock because of the death of his sister who died in a car accident. In the same accident his wife and brother were seriously injured. In family history his mother had cancer in 1958 and died after five months. The case was repertorised on Kent's Repertory as follows:

Grief, ailments from (p.51) + Clothes; Caust. Lach., Lyc., Nit.Ac., Nux.V., Puls.: loosening > (P.1348) +Tobacco < (P.1407). Lach., Lyc., Puls

+ Abdominal pain > by passing flatus (p.558) Lyc.

Lyc.,VI (i.e.6th potency of 50 millisimal scale) in water once a day with placebo given

10.5.63: Patient feels> pain nil: slight heaviness only – same medicine continued

02.9.63: Patient is much better but has a slight relapse – Medicine was repeated

Two years later I heard that he was well.

Case – 6:

Sri ESN aged 39 years turned up for consultation on 14–02–1963. He gets pain epigastrium < when hungry > after eating >eructation >pressure and > by bending forward. X ray report on 23–3-1961 showed Chronic duodenal ulcer. No other symptoms of value could be elicited. The case was reperterised – rice cause flatulence. He smokes 30 cigarettes a day from the last 7 years. He is outwardly calm and unperturbed but actually suppresses his feelings.

On 'Boger's Synoptic Key with the following symptoms.

Eating > (p.22) +Pressure >(p.27 + Bending > (p.19): Con. Ign. Plb. Sep. – – --Sepia 200 – 3 doses in one day and placebo given

07–3-63: finds very slight improvement – **Sep 1M – 3 doses** thrice in one day given.

14–3-63: Feels better, but gets pain when hungry – **Sep.VI (6th potency of 50 millisemal)** 1 dose daily to be taken in water.

21.3.63: He gets more pain with the medicine – **Sepia-200 – 3** doses in one day and placebo given. **As he felt better, medicine was repeated every week.**

18-4-63: Pain nil in day time, because he taken some food every 3 hours but gets pain at about 2 a.m. – Sepia 1M 3 doses in 1 day and placebo given.

03.5.63: Condition is same except intensity of pain which is reduced. Medicine was repeated.

09.5.63: Feels better but still gets pain at night. Sepia 10M – 3 doses in one day and Placebo.

25.5.63: Had slight pain through out the week – Sepia 50M – 3 doses in one day and placebo

06.6.63: Still gets pain – Sepia 3 four doses – twice a day given – 11.6.63: No improvement – Dys.Co. 12(bowel Nosode)– seven doses once a day given –No improvement even after repetition and off upto 25–12–63.

25–12–63: Kali bich: – better for 3 months:

23–03–64: Sepia 200 – twice a day

13–06–64: Completely relievd

CASES TREATED BY Y DR.P.C. MEHTA

To us the term peptic ulcer like the terms denoting all other diseases, is merely a diagnostic label and no more term has been given to it simply for the purpose of identification from other diseases and for pathologic classification. For us it is the individual, suffering from the disease, who is the focus of our attention and who needs our professional help. In the following series of cases, it will be seen that though the nosological diagnosis of the disease is same, every case was an individual case having its own peculiarities to be studied and treated on its own merits. This is the specialty of homoeopathy. Now I proceed with the cases diagnosed clinically as peptic ulcers.

Case – 1:

Some years ago, I was called in at 4 a.m. to see Mrs. B aged 48: who had suddenly vomited blood that morning, without any warming except for a complaint of some sore dragging feeling in the stomach previously. Her whole family was in a great alarm as they felt "she was bleeding to death". The blood was undoubtedly of gastric origin, having been vomited and with no evidence, past or present of lung disease. But for slight tenderness in the epigastrium there was practically no other sign or symptom. Because of the nature of the blood vomiting and the varicose veins the patient had, **Hemamalis 3**, in liquid form was prescribed every two hours with complete bed rest and abstinence for food. The patient was kept under observation. By next day, about 30 hours after that haemorrhage, the case was studied up again and **Acid Carbolic 30, 6 hourly, for two days was prescribed**. This remedy was of a very nervous temperament and she used to suffer from nervous dyspepsia of intensely painful character causing flatulent distension of abdomen with eructations and her discharges menstrual and lecuorrhoeh, were very putrid and corroding. Since then there has been no return of bleeding. After a few days of liquid nurishment, light solids were commenced. I was in touch with the case from time to time and she progressed well.

Case – 2:

A lady aged 28, 2 ½ months pregnant, quite fatty, fair complexioned consulted me for her gastric pains and dyspeptic symptoms which had existed for some time but had recently assumed an acute form. She had been under some local allopathic doctor's treatment which had failed to give relief. **Peptic ulcer was suspected.** On visitng her, I found that the **pain experienced was of an intensely screwing character spreading outwards from a point the size of small con, below the ensiform cartilage, felt through to the back.** Food of any kind, even liquids excited pains within 5 minutes of its ingestion, though temporary relief was felt during the actual meals. Relief was also experienced by heat. There was a history of rheumatic pains of erratic wandering nature. Great distress was felt from distension of the stomach which was not relieved by eructations. Epigastric tenderness was marked. The vomiting was of glairy, stringy mucus but no hameteosis or melaena. Thanks to homoeopathy, applied in the form of **Kali bich 30 in liquid form** given **3 hourly**, relief to the main symptoms followed in a few hours. The intensity of the pain became rapidly relieved and in the course of a day or two changed to a more drawing character with tendency to pass through to the back. **It entirely ceased in 5 days and the digestion became perfect for all intents and purposes.** Slight nausea, which was present from time to time was obviously due to pregnancy. She went to term and successfully delivered. I can vouch for the fact that she has never had any recurrence of the trouble for a pretty long time.

Case – 3:

A lady aged 42, of medium dark complexion, cheerful disposition called on me for consultation with a history of 7 years stomach pain which had become more intense for the last three weeks. Burning and constricting pains had developed and vomiting had occurred on several occasions in the previous week. Recently also she had often **passed per rectum bright red blood** as **much as a tea-spoonful a time. Stools were very dark at times black.** She was subject to diarrhoea in the past and for the past 3 to 4 days, she had as many 5 to 6 stools a day with sudden pasty stools with lot of burning in anus afterwards. **There was fissure at anus oozing offensive moisture. Pains** were felt from **right to left and considerable flatulent distension** was marked. Hot flushes and faintness accompanied the pain and she had actually fainted on few occasions. Tongue white coated. Examination elicited marked tenderness over the epigastrium especially to the left of the median line but there was no tenderness or lump. I restricted her to liquid diet and prescribed **Ferr. Phos 3x and after** that **Paenoia off. 3** repeatedly. A week latter the report was quite satisfactory, retching had stopped. Diarrhoea not so marked. A week later the report was quite satisfactory, retching was stopped. Diarrhoea not so marked. Malaena had been present on 3 occaisons but not for the last three days. She could not retain food comprising boiled eggs and porridge. The acute pains had now diminished to a mere discomfort in the pit of the stomach and flatulence was less. The medicine was continued in infrequent doses. The peculiar aspect of the case was that she had no periods for the last 3 days but now they returned to the great relief of the patient. After this she did not have the return of the trouble; of course the anal symptoms remained with much less intensity. She had regular menses and continued to enjoy excellent health (**Paeonia belongs to the order of the Puls.**)

Case – 4:

Another equally interesting case was of a lady, aged 32 who came to my clinic in great distress, disappointed with the three operations she had on the stomach and duodenum for recurring ulcers and the necessity for yet another one was felt necessary as she informed to save her life. The digestive disorder had commenced five years earlier with the help of X ray. An operation was performed and a suspicious looking appendix was also removed. Though she made a fairly quick recovery, there was no ultimate benefit and she felt very ill a year later. A second X ray examination was carried out as advised by another surgeon who arrived at the conclusion that the first operation had been a faulty one. So latter on a gastro-enterostomy was performed, at which an ulceration part of the tract of the length of a finger was removed but alas, with no better results so far as patient's general health was concerned. She developed an acute dread of the 4th operation which was now advised and then on she took a very pessimistic view of her future.

Her symptoms were flatulent dyspepsia with the violent attacks of burning pain with a sensation of boiling lead in the stomach. Annoying pain was experienced in the back and extreme lassitude rendering it impossible for her to perform her household duties. She had very offensive breath and she was constipated. Milk used to cause diarrhoea. Her diet was mainly of liquids. I **found tenderness over the epigastrium. Acid Carbolic 30** was prescribed in daily doses at first and later once every 3rd day, and after a fortnight that sensation of boiling lead in the stomach was less but expressed herself to be very much better. She could now attend to the household work. There was progressive improvement and the remedy was continued with breaks. **Later on some retroversion was corrected by Sepia** which also helped the general neurasthenic symptoms. When I saw her last, condition was: Except for an occasional slight sore feeling of the epigastrium, **all gastric symptoms had vanished. There was no tenderness in the epigastrium.** She could do a whole day's work at home without fatigue. A very peculiar thing and a great sign of improvement she could now do so and her hair which had become gray during her illness was now regaining its natural colour at the roots. Finally she declared "I do not remember over having feel so well in my whole life as I do now."

Case – 5:

The patient is a Marine Engineer in the Merchant Navy. **He went astray during a tour abroad and got an attack of gonorrhoea.** He suffered till he reached Bombay. Then he consulted a physician and took treatment but continued to suffer from **burning in the urethral meatus whenever there was the least dietetic error.** A few months latter thanks to allopathic treatment, he was free from his sensation. But later on he developed new symptoms and this was diagnosed as duodenal ulcer. He had burning pain in the epigastrium relieved by eating. **He took treatment in various places without any relief. On 25ᵗʰ Oct. 1967 he consulted me.** When I went into the case, **I decided that suppression of gonorrhoea was the cause.** As Dr. Phillip Rice has said in his book the cause and cure of Homoeopathic III, Hahnemann in para 8 of the Organaon, wrote the word "Zuffale" which meant totality of causes and casual events but according to him (Dr. Rice) Dr. Dudgeon wrongly interpreted and gave the sense as totality of symptoms. **So in this case the root cause was considered and by the administration of Thuja in different potencies we achieved very good results** – On the response of the gastric symptoms, the burning in the urethral orifice appeared again and the doctors on his ship diagnosed it is a case specific urethritis. But as this was a return of the previous symptoms about which the patient had been already advised he paid no attention and took no medicines. He became well and is still in touch with me. He is married and is enjoying normal health.

CHAPTER - 10

GERIATRIC – AILMENTS

DIET AND AGING

Relatively little is known about how the nutritional needs of older people differ from those who are younger. Although many people enjoy a generally healthy and vital old age, **age-related health problems do increase with advancing years and often have an effect on eating habits**

The science of gerontology, or the study of normal aging, is still quite new, and science is giving us new insights into aspects of aging that in the past have been accepted as "normal." While there is a similar pattern of changes that takes place among all humans as they age, these changes can occur at different rates in different individuals. We do not know how much of this difference is due to genetic make-up, and how much is due to lifestyle factors such as diet.

There is abundant evidence to show that an optimal level of nutrition can extend the lifespan and improve the quality of life. A large body of research examining the health of vegetarians, who typically consume a diet that is lower in calories, saturated fat, and protein, and higher in fiber and phytochemicals than nonvegetarians, shows that vegetarians suffer from less heart disease, obesity, high blood pressure, diabetes, and some forms of cancer. Vegetarians also tend to live longer than nonvegetarians.

Good eating habits throughout life can help to promote physical and mental well-being. For older people, eating right can help to minimize the symptoms of age-related changes that, for some, can cause discomfort or inconvenience. Although the aging process affects some people differently from others, everyone can benefit from eating a well-planned vegetarian diet.

Do Seniors Have Special Nutritional Needs?

Very little is known about how the aging process affects the body's ability to digest, absorb, and retain nutrients such as protein, vitamins, and minerals. Therefore, little is known about how the nutritional needs of older people differ from those of younger adults. Recommended nutrient intakes for seniors are currently extrapolated from those of younger adults, **one point that is generally agreed upon, however,** is that older people tend to take in less energy, or calories, than younger people. This may be due, in part, to a natural decline in the rate of metabolism as people age. It may also reflect a decrease in physical activity. If the total intake of food decreases, it follows that intakes of protein, carbohydrate, fat, vitamins, and minerals also decrease. If calorie intake is too low, then intakes of necessary nutrients may also be low.

Many other factors can affect the nutritional needs of older people and how successfully they meet those needs, including their access to food. For instance, some of the changes that take place as people age can affect the kinds of foods they can tolerate, and some can affect their ability to shop for or prepare food. As people age, problems such as high blood pressure or diabetes become more common, necessitating certain dietary modifications. Digestive system problems become more common, and some people may have trouble chewing or swallowing.

What Food one should Prefer?

Generally, current dietary recommendations for adults also apply to older people. The answer for this may be whatever that is fitting/

suiting to one consumed till today can be continued depending upon the **present** stage of the Digestive Tract or its ailments, life style, habits, and especially the financial state or any other problems

Author found frequently the following Ailments in the Aged

Physical – mental – environment problems, may affect more on old people than the present health problems for which suitable remedies could be given so as to expect some relief. Generally the first category of complaints may affect more than the actual Health problems, though the first category almost similar in young

Digestive Tract Remedies – Bio-chemic remedies agains – Different Ailments Remedies mentioned earlier are similar to all – Except the undernoted Other Remedies against different ailments in old people are as under:

DIGESTIVE TRACT REMEDIES – (30 potency as otherwise stated)	
Anacardium (Before meals)	Plug Sensation at Rectum – Apt to choke when eating or drinking. Swallows and drinks hastily. Abdomen Pain as if as if dull plug were pressed into intestines. Rumbling, pinching, griping. Rectum: Ineffectual desire, rectum seems powerless, as if plugged up. Bowels inactive. Spasmodic constriction of sphincture ani; even soft stool passes with difficulty. Itching at anus. Painful haemorrhoids.
Arg.Nit	Desire, craving for Sweets – Neurotic complaint – Brain and spinal symptoms presenting; themselves give certain indications for its homoeopathic employment. Symptoms of inco-ordination, loss of control and want of balance everywhere, mentally and physically. Nervous Dyspepsia – Hyperacidity – violent inflammation of the throat, and a marked gatro-enteritis ailments – **Pains increase and decrease gradually** – Headache with coldness and trembling Brain-fag. Titeness in Abdomen

Continued...

Canth, Nux-Vom., China	Indigestion-burning pain – cardiac region and flatulence – Go through each remedy and use the one covering the particular symptom i.e. burning sensation fitting in –only one dose weekly once – say for 3 weeks – when relief is there stop
Condurango	Constant burning sensation at ardiac orifice of stomach.
Catharis 30	Burning sensation of entire digestive Tract from stomach to Rectum with frequent urination > by rubbing – warm applications
Hydrastris 6 – Carbo. veg. Nux-vom.	Any one remedy to be used depending upon the results Dyspepsia in aged **out of which Hydrastis appears to act more more effectually** – 10 minutes before break-fast/ Lunch/dinner (Bio-chemic remedies comb.2) to improve digestion
Iris-vers	Mostly burning sensations right from throat to Anus through intestinal canal– Increase of sugar in blood due to Pancreatic Gland mal-function – relieved the entire complaint – also a **good** remedy for **diabetes** – Also **works on** thyroid, salivary, intestinal glands and especially gastro-intestinal mucous membrane are especially affected. – sore Liver – Diarrhoea.
Iris-vers	Mostly burning sensations right from throat to Anus through intestinal canal– Increase of sugar in blood due to Pancreatic Gland mal-function – relieved the entire complaint – also a **good** remedy for **diabetes** – Also **works on** thyroid, salivary, intestinal glands and especially gastro-intestinal mucous membrane are especially affected. – sore Liver – Diarrhoea –
Lycopodium (one dose at 8AM) once in a month.	Gastric symptoms passing stools in pieces – inguinal hernia more right side – hiatic hernia swith ifficulty in breathing – with biochemic also constipation even soft tool is – remedy Nat Phos. 6x to reduce hyperacidity

Nux-Mosch.	Bloating of stomach soon after eating – Constant Sleepy/ morose tendency through out day time, constipation – difficulty in breathing.

Miscellaneous Complaints – Remedies	
Chemomilla	Supressed or sudden Anger, irritation thereby trembling of the body
Glonoinum	Sun strokes of any age but especially for old people
Ignatia	For any shocks/loss of kith and kin or
Nux-Vomica	Often very irritative nature
Pulasitilla	Disturbed very with tears from eyes – especially women remedy – when pointed even when they are not the route cause for an incident. Changiable moods
Passiflora Q (Mother tincture)	When affected with an incident/too much disturbed/brain fag/pains due to accident, thereby sleeplessness may occur – a goody remedy for sleeplessness because of present day incidents stated or generally affected with that trouble – **It is a safe remedy** for disturbed sleep – and not habit forming. Especially this is the case of old people. (Dose10 drops in one ounce water)
Rhus-tox	Drenching in rain; *habituated more with cold water* daily head-bath/irrespective of age. Etc. for performing daily rituals especially are affected with Headaches, cold, at times fevers, body pains

GERIATRIC BYCO REMEDIES (COMBINATIONS) at 4 tablets – 3 times Per day – i.e. Break-fast – Lunch & Dinner – per fortnight – with week days gap for three months in all complaints except the one mentioned in conjunction with the Digestive Tract

Byco No	Nature of complaint	Combination of
02	Asthama	CP 3x, FP 3X, NM 6S, NS 3X
04	Constipation.	CP 3X, CF 3X, KM3X, NM 3X, SIL.6X
07	Diabetes	CP 3X, FP 3X, KP 3X, NP 3X, ND 6X
12	Headache	FP 3X, KP 3X, MP 3X, NM 3X
16	Nervous Exhaustion	CP 3X, FP 3X, KP 6X, MP 3X, NM 3X

Continued...

Byco No	Nature of complaint	Combination of
19	Rheumatism	CP 3X, FP 3X, KS 3X, MP 3X, NS 6X
25	Acidity, Flatulence & Indigestion	NP 3X, NS 6X, SIL 12X

ABREVIATIONS ADDRESSED

CF – Calcarea Fluor	KM – Kali Mur	NM – Natrum Mur
CP – Calcarea Phos	KP – Kali Phos	NP – Natrum Phos
CS – Calcarea Sulph	KS – Kali Sulph	NS – Natrum Sulph
FP – Ferrum Phos	MP – Magnesia Phos	Sil – Silicea

REFERENCE BOOKS/SOURCE

Sl.No	REFERENCE BOOKS	AUTHOR/SOURCE
01	A text book of Gynaecology	A.C. Cowperthaite
02	Anatomy and Physiology	Evylin Pierce
03	Chronic diseases its cause and cure	P.N. Bannerjee
04	Savill's Clinical Medicine	E.C. Warner
05	Children type	Doughlas M.Borland
06	Diseases of the Heart	A.L. Blackwood
07	Diseases of the Heart	Edwin M. Hale
08	Food tract and its ailments	A. L. Blackwood
09	Lectures on Homoeopathic Philosophy	James Tyler Kent
10	Materia Medica	Clarke
11	Materia Medica and guiding symptoms	Constantine Hering – M.D.
12	New Manual of Homoeopathic Materia Medica & Repertory (Revised edition 2000)	William Boericke
13	The twelve tissue remedies of Schussler:	William Boericke & Willis A. Duewey
14	Therapeutics	Samuel Lilienthal
15	Therapeutic-wise – Symptom/body part – wise arranged alphabetically	Dr. S.R. Pathak Dictionary
16	Homoeopathic Therapeutics	Samuel Liliental

Continued...

17	Select your Remedy	Rai Bahadur Bhishamber Das
18	Indian Journals of Homoeopathy from time to time	
19	https://en.wikibooks.org/wiki/HumanPhysiology/The gastrointestinal_ system	
20	Unabridged Dictionary Of The Senations "As If" – By James illium Ward – 2 Parts	

ABOUT THE AUTHOR

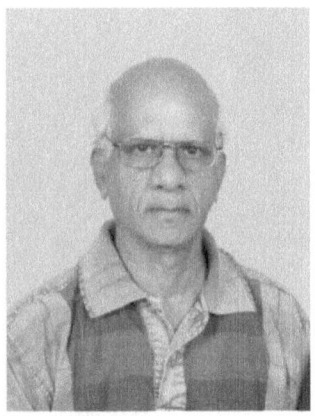

J V Mallapa Raju – Practicing Homoeopathy for more than 35 years.

He devoted all his time and acquired knowledge by constant study and practice. During his journey in Practicing, he had an opportunity to work with a different set of people with various difficulties. He was very instrumental in helping them with their ailments.

Of his earlier publishing were 'Lessons on Homoeopathy' and 'Handbook for Homoeopathy' with detailed information right from Basics to therapeutics of seasonal, paedaetric Complaints – Acute and Chronic, brief introduction to Anatomy & physiology.

Current book is a deep dive further into the body anatomy where he is covering details of **Digestive Tract** and problems/solutions relating to it.

The Future Releases will elaborate on other parts of the Human body and their Homoeopathy remedies, it will also cover detailed information on how to deal chronic ailments pertaining to them. Mainly covering the ailments of Arthritis, Rheumatic Complaints, skin ailments, Pediatric, and on Gynics.

He wish to extend online medical advice through mails and he can be reached at jvmraju@gmail.com. Person reaching out would need to send his/her entire case history attached with respective scanned copies of reports, if any.

ABOUT THE BOOK

Details of "Handbook For Homoeopathy"

On Common ailments written by the Author Mr. Raju are as under.

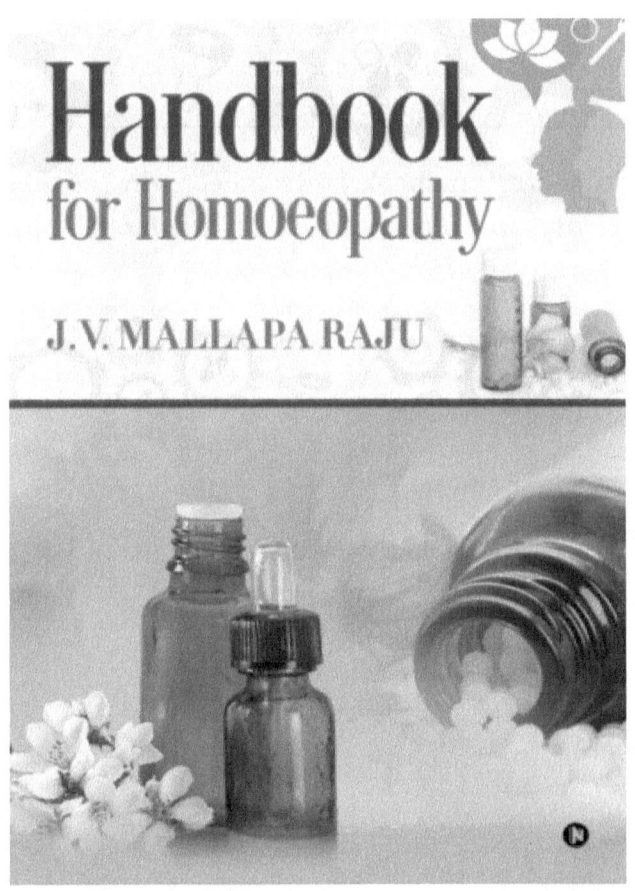

It gives details right from the basics to principles and treatment of common ailments with Homoeo Remedies.

CONTENTS: Brief History – Introduction of laws of Homoeopathy – How the Homoeo remedies are prepared & materials used for their preparations – Evaluation of symptoms and their importance – Different ways of finding a remedy – Treatment of common ailments with names of remedies i.e. (a) Digestive complaints in short (b) Urinary Tract (c) Headache (d) Aches & Pains i.e. right from top to bottom (e) Respiratory Tract (f) Fevers (g) Emergencies accidents like fractures, concussions/burns, injuries etc (h) Skin diseases (i) Heart and Circulatory system (j) Diseases peculiar to women (k) Children type – remedies basing on Behaviour, body get up – likes & Dislikes, interest on studies, and on their ailments in brief

A list of Polychrest remedies, frequently indicated (50 Nos) given in the book may be stored in a closed wooden/card board box – The names of books written by Eminent Authors are also noted under each Chapter.

Printed edition of " Handbook for Homoeopathy" could be ordered through – *amazon.in – flipkar.com and infbeam.com*

www.ingramcontent.com/pod-product-compliance
Lightning Source LLC
Chambersburg PA
CBHW030609220526
45463CB00004B/1228